# Touch Therapy

2

13

Wc

*For Churchill Livingstone:*

*Senior Commissioning Editor:* Inta Ozols
*Project Development Manager:* Valerie Dearing
*Project Manager:* Jane Shanks

# Touch Therapy

**Tiffany Field** PhD
Director, Touch Research Institutes, University of Miami School of Medicine and
Nova Southeastern University, Florida, USA

Foreword by
**Leon Chaitow** ND DO
Practitioner and Senior Lecturer, Centre for Community Care and
Primary Health, University of Westminster, London, UK

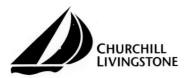

CHURCHILL
LIVINGSTONE

EDINBURGH LONDON NEW YORK OXFORD PHILADELPHIA ST LOUIS SYDNEY TORONTO 2000

CHURCHILL LIVINGSTONE
An imprint of Elsevier Limited

First published 2000
  Reprinted 2003 (twice), 2005

ISBN 0 443 05791 5

**British Library Cataloguing in Publication Data**
A catalogue record for this book is available from the British Library

**Library of Congress Cataloging in Publication Data**
A catalog record for this book is available from the Library of Congress

your source for books,
journals and multimedia
in the health sciences
**www.elsevierhealth.com**

The
publisher's
policy is to use
paper manufactured
from sustainable forests

Printed in China
B/04

# Contents

# Foreword

Massage has been practiced world wide, in a variety of styles, for many centuries, and is well accepted by the public at large as being pleasant, relaxing and safe. However, until recently there has been a dearth of well designed, controlled studies to validate its potential to offer real therapeutic benefit to people in states of ill health and dysfunction. One of the principal requirements of modern health care provision can be summed up by the term, 'evidence based'. It is no longer sufficient for any therapeutic approach to simply rely on a long history of use, or popularity, or widespread availability, to justify its continued acceptance (especially if insurance reimbursement is anticipated). Official licensing agencies, insurance companies, medical authorities, and an increasingly demanding media and public, require evidence of both safety and efficacy, of all forms of therapeutic intervention.

As the historical trend towards integration between complementary and mainstream health care evolves at a steadily increasing pace, complementary methods (and few methods are more 'complementary' than massage) are being scrutinized with demands for documented evidence that they work, are safe, and can readily be combined with other therapeutic approaches. To meet this need, and in a search for explanations of the mechanisms involved in achieving the benefits observed, the Touch Research Institutes, under the direction of Tiffany Field, has undertaken the task of investigating the effects of standardized massage application in a wide array of conditions, and this book describes many of these studies. Whether states of dysfunction or ill health have causes which are biomechanical, psychosocial, biochemical, or – as is likely – a combination of these elements, massage seems to be able to exert a beneficial influence. Biomechanically, tissues can be stretched, relaxed and mobilized, while circulation is simultaneously improved and drainage enhanced. Psychosocially massage exerts its influence on the individual's perception of anxiety and 'tension', allowing more specific approaches to deal with underlying causes. Biochemically, as many of the studies reported on in the book attest, significant changes occur in, for example, stress hormone levels. As long as therapeutic interventions are performing a role in which they reduce the adaptive burden to which the individual is responding, or improve those functions which are stressed by the adaptive processes, a positive contribution can be seen to be being made towards a healthier state.

Massage, it seems, performs just such services irrespective of whether the focus is preterm infants, and the potential for enhancing their growth and wellbeing; reduction in pain (in a variety of situations ranging from burn patients to PMS, childbirth, fibromyalgia and headaches); reduction in intensity of the symptoms of anxiety or depression; beneficial modulation of symptoms in autoimmune conditions, as well as enhancement of immune function, massage is shown to offer a range of benefits, in an incredibly varied series of well conducted studies. Interestingly, in some studies, positive effects were shown to accrue to those giving the massage, for example when grandparents massage their grandchildren.

This book will deservedly become a major resource for all therapists involved in bodywork (not only massage therapists), and for all those teaching massage therapy in particular, and bodywork in general. In particular it should be read by anyone considering employing, or referring patients to, a massage therapist, so that they can become familiar with what is possible, and what can be expected, when they do so.

Teaching and professional organizations responsible for massage therapy, and those active as massage therapists, have the obligation to their profession, as well as to the public, to ensure that the standards of education, continuing professional development, and practice, match the potential which Tiffany Field has so diligently laid before us in this book.

London, 1999                                                    Leon Chaitow

# Acknowledgements

I would like to acknowledge all the patients, therapists and researchers who participated in these studies. Johnson and Johnson and the National Institutes of Health were also instrumental in funding this research for which we are very grateful.

1999                                                              Tiffany Field

# Introduction

Touch therapy is one of the oldest forms of treatment in the world, having first been described in China during the second century BC and soon after in India and Egypt. Hippocrates, in 400 BC, defined medicine as 'the art of rubbing.' Massage therapy disappeared from the American medical scene at approximately the time of the pharmaceutical revolution of the 1940s. Now considered an 'alternative' therapy, it is becoming popular again as part of the alternative medicine movement. At this time, it is commonly defined by massage therapists as the manipulation of soft tissue by trained therapists for therapeutic purposes. Despite its long history and popularity, a MEDLINE search yielded only approximately 200 articles from the last 30 years. Much of this literature suffers from classic methodological problems. First, although the literature has focused on clinical conditions, very few studies are based on clinical trials. Typical sampling problems are the failure to include control groups and the lack of random assignment to treatment and control conditions. Often, the subjects have served as their own controls and the measures were simply collected at the beginning and the end of the treatment period. Although within-individual controls are important in controlling for individual differences, treatment individuals need to be compared with non-treatment or comparison treatment individuals. Using a within-subjects design alone could result in effects that might be explained otherwise by spontaneous recovery, a placebo effect or statistical regression. The control group would optimally be an attention control or a comparison treatment control to avoid the possibility that the therapist's attention alone explained the effects.

A second problem is the very small sample sizes used in most of the studies, and the treatment group often receiving more than one type of treatment. Another problem is the potential for initial level effects where the treatment may have differential effects depending on the initial level of the subjects. This, in itself, could explain many of the mixed findings. Still another problem is the use of inappropriate statistics. Only two meta-analyses appear in the literature. This has occurred because there are not enough studies with comparable designs and standards, and too many different massage therapy techniques have been used across the studies. Very few replications and virtually no follow-up studies have been conducted. Although one might not expect massage therapy to have sustained effects any more than temporary drugs, diet or exercise, follow-ups are needed to assess that question. Finally, there would appear to be a publication bias where, inevitably, positive results are published and negative results lie idle.

For the above reasons, we have conducted a number of massage therapy studies focusing on a variety of different conditions that might benefit from massage therapy. In each of these studies there was a theoretical reason to expect positive results. In addition, other studies from the literature are included in this review if they meet the criteria of adequate sample size based on power analysis and random assignment to treatment and/or a comparison treatment or an attention control group.

The massage therapy technique used throughout all of these studies, unless otherwise specified, involved deep tissue manipulation with presumed stimulation of pressure receptors. All adult studies involved eight sessions (two per week for four consecutive weeks) of 30 minutes' duration, and all child sessions were performed by parents on a nightly basis for 30 days for 15 minutes' duration. The parameters for the adult sessions were based on practical considerations, namely that most adults could not afford more than two half-hour sessions per week by a professional or by a significant other. The parameters of the child sessions were based on the consideration that children with chronic illness may benefit from a 'daily dose' and that their parents could also benefit from providing the massage at no monetary expense to themselves.

The studies are grouped thematically by the primary objective of treatment: for example, facilitating growth or reducing pain. They are organized in a sequence that may seem arbitrary but one that seems to capture the longitudinal progression from primary agendas early in life to those later in life: for example, focusing on facilitating growth in premature infants, for the early life agenda, to enhancing immune function, a more primary agenda for later in life. An attempt is made throughout to address potential underlying mechanisms that are unique to the different conditions as well as to discuss an overarching potential mechanism for massage therapy across conditions. Thus, the order selected is facilitating growth, pain reduction, increasing alertness, diminishing stress, anxiety and depression, and enhancing immune function.

This book is a review of research on touch therapy conducted at the Touch Research Institutes. Hopefully it will be helpful to those who are interested in touch as a form of therapy and touch therapy research.

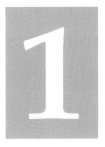

# Enhancing growth

## ANIMAL MODELS

Data from research on rats and monkeys support the use of touch as therapy for enhancing growth. In a model developed by Saul Schanberg, Cynthia Kuhn, and colleagues, rat pups were first removed from their mother to investigate touch deprivation. In several studies a decrease was noted in growth hormone (ornithine decarboxylase) when the pups were removed from their mother (Schanberg & Field 1987). This decrease was observed in all body organs, including heart, liver, and brain, and in all parts of the brain, including the cerebrum, cerebellum and brain stem. These values returned to normal when the pups were stimulated using techniques approximating the mother's behavior. Observations were made of rat mothers' nocturnal behavior; they frequently tongue licked, pinched, and carried around the rat pups. When the researchers tried each of these maneuvers, only the tongue licking (simulated by a paint brush dipped in water and briskly stroked all over the body of the rat pup) restored the growth hormone values to their normal level, suggesting that pressure or stimulation of pressure receptors is critical for facilitating growth. More recently, Schanberg and his colleagues discovered a gene that is triggered by touch, leading to protein synthesis, suggesting genetic origins of this touch–growth relationship (Schanberg 1995).

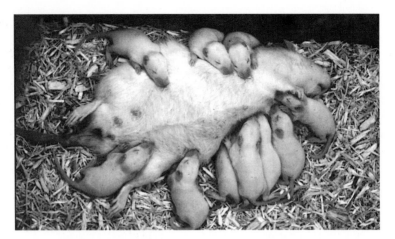

**Figure 1.1**   Anesthetized mother rat and her touch-deprived pups.

Related studies by Meaney (Meaney et al 1990) and colleagues suggest a long-term impact of handling for the reduction of cortisol (stress hormone) production. Rats who were handled more as pups showed less corticosteroid production, more elaborate dendritic arborization in the hippocampal region, and better maze performance (memory function) in the aging rat.

## PRETERM INFANTS

Parallels have been noted in human infants. At the Hammersmith Hospital in London, Modi, Glover, and colleagues (Acolet et al 1993) conducted studies showing cortisol reduction in preterm infants who were being massaged. The biochemical and clinical response to massage in preterm infants was assessed. Eleven stable infants, of 29 weeks median gestational age, median birth weight 980 g, and median postnatal age 20 days, were studied. Blood samples were obtained for the determination of epinephrine, norepinephrine, and cortisol 45 minutes before the start of massage and approximately 1 hour after completion of massage. Cortisol, but not catecholamine, concentrations decreased consistently after massage. There was a slight decrease in skin temperature, but there was no change in oxygenation or oxygen requirement. This study showed that it is possible to detect an objective hormonal change following touch intervention in preterm infants. These authors are currently using magnetic resonance imaging with their massaged preterm infants to determine whether there is greater dendritic arborization of the hippocampal region, as in the rat data by Meaney et al (1990).

We have conducted several studies showing greater weight gain in preterm infants, including those who are cocaine-exposed (Wheeden et al 1993) and HIV-exposed (Scafidi & Field 1996). In those studies, massage with some pressure was used. Although infants, particularly premature infants, may seem to be fragile, some pressure is needed for the massage to be effective. In our review of the infant massage literature we found that those who used light stroking did not report weight gain, for example, whereas those who used stroking with pressure did report weight gain (Scafidi et al 1986). These studies are elaborated in the next sections.

In our studies on preterm newborns in the neonatal intensive care unit, the infants were given 15-minute massages three times a day for 10 days while they were still in the incubator (massaged through the incubator portholes) (Field et al 1986, Scafidi et al 1990). In the first study the treated infants compared with controls gained 47% more weight and were hospitalized for 6 days fewer. Today that would translate into a cost saving of $10 000 per infant. At that rate, 4.7 billion dollars in hospital costs could be saved per year by massaging the 470 000 preterm infants born each year! Elevated norepinephrine and epinephrine levels in these infants suggested that massage therapy was facilitating the normal developmental increase typically noted in these catecholamines at this beginning stage in life (Kuhn et al 1991). Finally, the treated infants performed better on the Brazelton Neonatal Behavior Assessment Scale. Their orientation scores were better, suggesting increased responsiveness to social stimulation, their motor behavior was more organized, and they received better habituation scores, suggesting that they learned more quickly to ignore an irrelevant stimulus (e.g. repeated soundings of a bell or buzzer). Eight months later they were still showing a weight gain advantage and were performing better on the Bayley Mental and Motor Scales (Field, Scafidi & Schanberg 1987). We speculated that this superior growth and development resulted from better parent–infant interactions that were facilitated by the infants being more responsive during the newborn period. This study and other studies on preterm infants exposed to other risk factors are reviewed in the following pages.

## Study 1: Tactile–kinesthetic stimulation (massage) effects on preterm newborns

In these studies we elected to follow the procedure that had been most effective in previous studies. It was called tactile–kinesthetic stimulation then because massage therapy was a term that was not being used in the pediatric literature. Unfortunately, most studies that preceded ours were ineffective, most likely because they used light stroking which was like a tickle stimulus and was aversive to the infants. We used deeper pressure because the infants behaved as if they preferred deeper pressure.

*Method*

**Sample** The sample included 40 preterm neonates from a neonatal intensive care unit (NICU) who fulfilled the following criteria:

1. gestational age < 36 weeks; birthweight < 1500 g
2. absence of congenital heart malformations, gastrointestinal disorders, CNS disturbances, congenital anomalies, and maternal drug addiction
3. weight upon admission to the transitional care nursery between 1100 and 1650 g.

Infants were admitted to the transitional care ('grower') nursery when they were considered medically stable and were no longer receiving oxygen supplementation or intravenous feedings. After the infants entered this nursery and informed consent had been obtained, they were randomly assigned to the treatment or control group based on a stratification of gestational age, birthweight, number of NICU days, and transitional care nursery admission weight. Based on nursery statistics from the previous year, we predicted that our NICU neonates would generally average 30 weeks gestational age, 1300 g birth weight, 30 NICU days, and 1400 g transitional nursery admission weight. We then used these averages as cutoff points to randomly assign infants to one of eight cells per group. Thus, each group featured the same number of infants who were either above or below the cutoff points on each of these four measures. As shown in Table 1.1, the treatment and control groups were equivalent on these and other birth measures.

**Procedure** Routine grower nursery procedures included feeding orders that were based on daily weight gain. The total intake of calories and the volume of each feeding was specified. Nippling and weaning from the isolette were initiated according to each infant's tolerance of the procedure. All neonates in the study were in isolettes and were bottle-fed for the duration of the study. Hospital discharge occurred at 1800 g if oral feeding, temperature maintenance, and metabolic regulation were adequate.

**Table 1.1**  Baseline neonatal measures[1] (Study 1)

| Measures | Stimulation group | | Control group | |
| --- | --- | --- | --- | --- |
| Gestational age (weeks) | 31 | (2.2) | 31 | (2.8) |
| Birth wt (g) | 1280 | (249) | 1268 | (199) |
| Birth length (cm) | 39 | (2.9) | 39 | (3.8) |
| Ponderal index | 2.2 | (0.3) | 2.2 | (0.3) |
| Head circumference at birth (cm) | 28 | (2.1) | 27 | (2.1) |
| Apgar (1 min) | 5.9 | (1.8) | 5.8 | (2.2) |
| Apgar (5 min) | 7.8 | (1.0) | 7.7 | (1.6) |
| Obstetric Complications Scale score | 87 | (17.1) | 86 | (13.6) |
| Postnatal Complications Scale score (neonatal intensive care unit) | 79 | (20.5) | 76 | (18.3) |
| Stay in neonatal intensive care unit | 20 | (4.5) | 20 | (4.0) |
| Wt at onset stimulation period | 1393 | (114) | 1385 | (131) |
| Postnatal Complications Scale score (transitional nursery) | 142 | (27.9) | 138 | (30.7) |

[1] Results are means with standard deviations in parentheses.

Each infant in the treatment group received tactile–kinesthetic stimulation for three 15-minute periods at the beginning of three consecutive hours starting at approximately 30 minutes after the first morning feeding) for 10 weekdays with a nontreatment weekend intervening. This schedule was used to approximate those stimulation schedules that had proven effective in previous studies (Rausch 1981, White & Labarba 1976). The 15-minute stimulation sessions consisted of three standardized 5 minute phases. Tactile stimulation was given during the first and third phases, and kinesthetic stimulation was given during the middle phase. For the tactile stimulation, the neonate was placed in a prone position. After thorough hand scrubbing, the person providing stimulation placed the palms of his or her warmed hands on the infant's body through the isolette portholes. He/she then gently stroked with his/her hands for five 1 minute periods (12 strokes at approximately 5 seconds per stroking motion) over each region in the following sequence:

1. from the top of the head to the neck and back again
2. from the neck across the shoulders and back again
3. from the upper back to the waist and back again
4. from the hip to the foot to the hip on both legs
5. from the shoulder to the hand to the shoulder on both arms.

The infant was then placed in a supine position for the subsequent kinesthetic stimulation phase. This phase contained five 1-minute segments of six passive flexion/extension movements (like bicycling) lasting approximately 10 seconds apiece for each arm, then each leg, and finally both legs together. The infant was then returned to a prone position for the final stimulation phase in which the procedure was repeated.

**Measures** Clinical data recorded from the hospital charts included daily weight, formula intake (volume and calories), frequency of voiding and stooling, average respiration rate, heart rate, and body temperature, number of apneic episodes, and parent visits. Obstetric and postnatal complication data were summarized on the Obstetric and Postnatal Complications Scales (Littman & Parmelee 1978).

Sleep/wake behavior observations were made for a 45-minute period at the beginning and end of the stimulation program (on day 1 and 10 at least 4 hours after the last stimulation session) using Thoman's criteria for sleep/wake states (Thoman 1975). Unlike the global state evaluations of neonatal neurologic examinations, the Thoman coding system involves recording state changes at frequent (10-second) intervals. In addition, the presence of body movements (limb, trunk, or head movements) was recorded at 10-second intervals during the sleep/wake observation period as a general measure of activity level. Finally, the Brazelton Neonatal Behavior Assessment Scale (Brazelton 1973) was administered at the end of the treatment period (day 12), and performance was summarized on the following dimensions: habituation, orientation, motor behavior, range of state, regulation of state, autonomic stability, and reflexes (Lester et al 1982). The researchers who conducted the sleep/wake behavior observations and the Brazelton assessments did not know (or were 'blind' to) the group assignments.

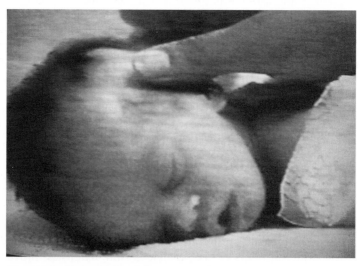

**Figure 1.2**  Preterm infant being massaged.

**Table 1.2**   Measures differentiating tactile–kinesthetic stimulation preterm neonates from control infants[1] (Study 1)

| Measures | Stimulation group | | Control group | | $p$ |
|---|---|---|---|---|---|
| Feedings (No./d)[2] | 8.6 | (1.3) | 9.0 | (1.3) | NS |
| Formula (mL/kg/d)[2] | 171.0 | (8.5) | 166.0 | (17.5) | NS |
| Calories/kg/d[2] | 114.0 | (5.7) | 112.0 | (12.2) | NS |
| Calories/d[2] | 169.0 | (11.2) | 165.0 | (27.1) | NS |
| Daily wt gain (g)[2] | 25.0 | (6.0) | 17.0 | (6.7) | 0.0005 |
| g/calorie/kg | 0.21 | (0.04) | 0.15 | (0.04) | 0.0005 |
| % time awake | 16.0 | (15.5) | 7.0 | (10.7) | 0.0005 |
| % time movement | 32.0 | (5.6) | 25.0 | (6.2) | 0.04 |
| Brazelton scores[3] | | | | | |
| Habituation | 6.1 | (0.6) | 4.9 | (0.5) | 0.02 |
| Orientation | 4.8 | (0.9) | 4.0 | (1.0) | 0.02 |
| Motor | 4.7 | (0.7) | 3.9 | (1.0) | 0.03 |
| Range of state | 4.6 | (0.8) | 3.9 | (1.0) | 0.03 |

[1] Results are means with standard deviations in parentheses.
[2] Means for these measures were derived from daily measures averaged across the 12-day treatment period.
[3] Higher scores are optimal. The range of scores for the stimulation and control groups, respectively, were as follows: Habituation, 5 to 7, 3 to 8; orientation, 3 to 7, 2 to 6; motor, 3 to 6, 2 to 6; range of state, 3 to 6, 2 to 6.

## Results

The data analyses revealed the following group differences (see Table 1.2).

1. The treatment infants averaged 8 g (47%) more weight gain per day than the control infants, even though the groups did not differ on number of feedings per day or average formula intake (volume or calories) either prior to or during the treatment period. Also, the treatment group gained more weight per calories of intake per kilogram of body weight. The mean daily weight gain for the treatment and control groups during the stimulation period is shown in Figure 1.3.

2. The treatment infants were awake (drowsy or alert inactivity) and active a greater percentage of time during the sleep/wake behavioral observations.

3. The treatment infants, as assessed by the Brazelton scale, showed more mature habituation, orientation, motor and range of state behavior.

4. The treatment infants were hospitalized 6 days fewer than the control infants after the onset of the treatment period (18.4 vs 24.7 days), yielding an average hospital cost savings of $3000 per infant in our hospital setting. Today, the equivalent cost savings would be $10 000 per infant.

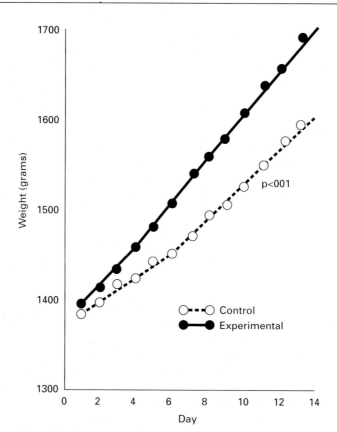

**Figure 1.3** Daily weight gain in massaged and control group preterm infants.

## Discussion

These data suggest that very small, preterm neonates benefit from tactile–kinesthetic stimulation administered during their stay in a transitional care nursery. The stimulation contributed to greater weight gain, increased motor activity, more alertness, and improved performance on the Brazelton scale. While the greater activity and alertness during sleep/wake observations and in turn the better Brazelton scale performance of the treatment infants could possibly result from stimulation that was received prior to these assessments, this is unlikely because at least 4 hours had intervened between the stimulation session and the assessments. Although the greater weight gain could be explained by differential treatment provided by the nurses who could not be unaware of the group assignments, this possibility is also unlikely inasmuch as nurses are more often noted to provide compensatory treatment for control infants than for intervention infants during stimulation studies (Field 1980,

Schaeffer, Hatcher & Barglow 1980). This type of differential treatment by the nurses would merely provide a more conservative test of the effectiveness of the stimulation program. It is also improbable that the treatment infants were initially more active, alert, and behaviorally mature and thus gained more weight, inasmuch as they did not differ from the control infants on several baseline measures (e.g., gestational age and birth weight) that typically correlate with behavioral maturity (Field 1980, Schaeffer et al 1980). Finally, these data are supported by other supplemental stimulation studies reporting greater weight gain, motor activity, and alertness in preterm neonates who did not require intensive care (Solkoff & Matuszak 1975, White & Labarba 1976), suggesting that these treatment effects may be robust despite these potential confounds. Nonetheless, future studies would desirably include baseline measures of behavior and activity as well as longer-term follow-up measures.

The mediating mechanisms for the greater weight gain of the stimulated neonates cannot be determined from these data. Formula intake was not a significant factor, because caloric consumption did not differ in the two groups. In addition, the groups did not differ on the amount of regurgitation, based on nurses' reports. Furthermore, caloric intake was not a significant factor in a study in which a similar form of stimulation (given to rat pups) effectively reversed maternal deprivation-associated decreases in growth hormone release and ornithine decarboxylase activity, which is known to be a sensitive index of tissue growth (Schanberg, Evoniuk & Kuhn 1984).

'Maternal deprivation' or inadequate stimulation may result in impaired metabolic efficiency. Our group comparisons indicate that the treatment infants gained more weight per calories of intake than the control group. This apparent increase in conversion of caloric intake to weight gain could be due to an alteration in basal metabolic function per se or to an increase in weight gain efficiency secondary to increased activity. Altered metabolic efficiency has been associated with activity level changes in rats (Mittleman & Valenstein 1984, Mussachia et al 1980) and in humans (Torun et al 1979, Young & Torun 1981). In addition, increased activity is associated with elevated growth hormone release in humans (VanWyk & Underwood 1978). Our data are consistent with those reported on 2- to 4-year-old malnourished children stimulated to be more physically active (Torun et al 1979, Young & Torun 1981). These stimulated children were more active and gained more weight per caloric intake than the control group despite equivalent caloric intake and a 30% greater caloric expenditure.

Inadequate stimulation appears to contribute to diminished activity and growth failure in maternally deprived rat pups (Schanberg, Evoniuk & Kuhn 1984), in nonorganic failure to thrive infants (Powell, Brasel & Blizzard 1967), and in preterm neonates, suggesting a potentially similar underlying physiologic mechanism. Longer recordings of sleep/wake behavior and activity level (i.e., 24-hour video recordings) would be desirable in future studies to determine whether the stimulated infants are consistently more active and alert. In addition, neuroendocrine measures (e.g., cortisol and catecholamines) and metabolic efficiency assessments (e.g., nitrogen balance) should provide informative data on the relationships between stimulation, motor activity, stress reduction, and weight gain.

The treatment neonates also showed better performance on the Brazelton scale, specifically in the areas of habituation, orientation, motor, and range of state behaviors. The greater alertness and motor activity of the treatment infants may have contributed to their more organized behavior on the subsequent Brazelton assessment. Better performance on the Brazelton scale may facilitate early parent–infant interactions which, in turn, may affect the later development of these preterm infants (Field, Dempsey & Shuman 1984). Finally, the shorter hospital stay, yielding significant cost savings, suggests that this may be a cost-effective intervention for small preterm neonates during their stay in transitional care nurseries.

### Replications of this study

A replication of this study was subsequently conducted by Scafidi et al 1990). Forty preterm infants (mean gestational age = 30 weeks; mean birth weight = 1176 g; mean duration ICU care = 14 days) were assigned to treatment and control groups once they were considered medically stable. Assignments were based on a random stratification of gestational age, birth weight, intensive care duration, and study entrance weight. The treatment infants ($N = 20$) received tactile–kinesthetic stimulation for three 15-minute periods during 3 consecutive hours per day for a 10-day period. Sleep/wake behavior was monitored and Brazelton assessments were performed at the beginning and at the end of the treatment period. The treated infants averaged a 21% greater weight gain per day (34 vs 28 g) and were discharged 5 days earlier. No significant differences were demonstrated in sleep/wake states and activity level between the groups. The treated infants' performance was superior on the habituation cluster items of the Brazelton scale.

Finally, the treatment infants were more active during the stimulation sessions than during the nonstimulation observation sessions (particularly during the tactile segments of the sessions). Although these data confirm the positive effects of tactile–kinesthetic stimulation, the underlying mechanisms remained unknown at this point.

In attempting to understand the mechanism underlying the relationship between massage therapy and weight gain, we conducted research in which we assessed vagal tone. The vagus (one of the twelve cranial nerves) slows the heart during tasks that require attention, and it enhances gastric motility and facilitates the release of food absorption hormones like insulin. Both vagal activity, as assessed by a vagal tone monitor (which transforms heart rate into vagal tone or the respiratory sinus arrhythmia component of heart rate), and insulin levels increased following the massage therapy (Scafidi et al 1996). The massaged infants did not eat more food, nor did they sleep more, so they were not simply conserving calories. Rather, the weight gain seems to have been mediated by an increase in vagal activity, which facilitated the release of food absorption hormones (at least insulin).

At 8 months the treated infants were still showing a weight advantage and they performed better on the Bayley Scales of Infant Development (Field et al 1987). On the mental scale their scores averaged 12 points higher and on the motor scale 13 points higher than the untreated infants. The infants' greater responsiveness, as assessed by the Brazelton Neonatal Behavior Assessment, apparently elicited more stimulation from their parents, which led to the later gains in growth and development.

## OTHER HIGH-RISK INFANTS

Other high-risk infants were being treated in the neonatal intensive care nursery whom we thought might also benefit from massage therapy: for example, infants exposed to cocaine and HIV-exposed newborns. Thus, we conducted the same massage therapy protocol with those groups of infants.

### Study 2: Cocaine-exposed infants

Similar weight gains were noted in our study on cocaine-exposed infants (Wheeden et al 1993). In addition, the massaged versus the nonmassaged infants showed superior motor behavior.

As had been shown in the previous studies, tactile–kinesthetic stimulation (massage) facilitates growth and development of healthy preterm infants (Barnard & Bee 1983; Ottenbacher et al

1987). Massaged preterm infants experienced greater weight gain, more mature awake and active behavior, and more mature motor activity (Field et al 1986, Scafidi et al 1986, Scafidi et al 1990).

Although these studies documented the benefits of massage on healthy preterm infants, nothing was known about those effects on preterm infants exposed to cocaine and other drugs in utero.

Cocaine-exposed newborns experienced more perinatal complications and neurological and behavioral abnormalities (Burkett, Yasin & Palow 1990, Coles et al 1990, Eisen et al 1991). The most frequent of these complications are spontaneous abortion, abruptio placentae, intrauterine growth retardation, premature birth, and decreased head circumference, birth weight, and length (Hadeed & Siegel 1989, Rosenak et al 1990). In addition to these complications, more subtle central nervous system deficits indicative of fetal distress have been noted, including lower vagal tone, increased heart rate, and lower Apgar scores (Richards, Kulkarni & Bremner 1990). Furthermore, behavioral studies have found a tendency for cocaine-exposed newborns to show more stress behaviors (tremor/clonus, restlessness, irritability, hypertonia, and abnormal reflexes) than do nonexposed infants (Eisen et al 1991). Because massage therapy is noted to facilitate weight gain and reduce stress behaviors in preterm newborns, that treatment may help cocaine-exposed preterm newborns. Thus, the aim of this study was to examine the therapeutic effects of massage on the growth and development of preterm cocaine-exposed neonates.

### Method

**Sample** The sample was comprised of 30 preterm cocaine-exposed neonates from an intermediate care unit. Criteria for inclusion in the study were:

1. gestational age < 37 weeks as determined by the Dubowitz Scale (Dubowitz, Dubowitz & Goldberg 1970)
2. birth weight < 1500 g
3. no genetic anomalies, chromosomal aberrations, congenital heart malformations, gastrointestinal disturbances, overt manifestations of congenital infection or maternal seropositivity for syphilis, hepatitis B, or human immunodeficiency virus, nor central nervous system dysfunctions
4. a neonatal intensive care unit duration of < 50 days
5. an entry weight into the study between 1000 and 1650 g
6. a positive urine or meconium toxicology screen or a positive maternal self-report for cocaine.

Although it would have been desirable to eliminate infants who also had been exposed to alcohol, tobacco, or marijuana, past studies show that as many as 85% of our drug-exposed newborns are polydrug exposed (Eisen et al 1991). Thus, although the focus of this study was on cocaine-exposed neonates, it might be more accurate to refer to these infants as polydrug-exposed neonates. Despite the polydrug nature of the population, cocaine was the primary drug reported in the sample. Neonates were not eligible for the study until they were considered medically stable, were free from ventilatory assistance and were receiving no intravenous medications or feedings. The cocaine-exposed neonates were assigned to the treatment (massage) or control (no massage) groups based on a random stratification procedure to ensure equivalence between groups on gestational age, birth weight, intensive care unit duration, and entry weight into the study.

**Procedure** During this study all infants continued to receive standard nursery care including: (1) daily examination by a physician; (2) feeding by a nurse, nurse's assistant, or 'grandmother' volunteer, and (3) weaning from the isolette at 1700 g. Infants were discharged at a weight of 1800 g contingent on self-regulation of temperature and metabolites. In accord with hospital protocol, parents were encouraged to visit, hold, and feed their infants.

Massage therapy was provided for 15 of the cocaine-exposed infants for three 15-minute periods during 3 consecutive hours each day for a 10-day period. The 15-minute stimulation session was comprised of three standardized 5-minute phases. The first and third phases were stroking different body parts (tactile stimulation), whereas the middle phase was moving the upper and lower limbs into flexion and extension (kinesthetic stimulation). This massage therapy was the same procedure used in our previous massage studies (Study 1, this chapter), thus allowing comparison across samples and studies. All massage therapy sessions were conducted by the same research assistant trained in the procedure.

**Measures** Data were recorded daily from the nursing notes, including:

1. daily weight
2. volumetric and caloric intake
3. number of feedings
4. frequency of urination and stooling
5. average respiration rate, heart rate, and body temperature
6. number of apneic episodes
7. parental visits, including touching, holding, and feeding by the parents or caregiver.

The Obstetric Complications Scale (OCS) (Littman & Parmelee 1978), The Postnatal Complications Scale (PCS) (Littman & Parmelee 1978), the Newfoundland Scale (Scheiner & Sexton 1991) (consisting of 18 complications weighted on a four-point scale according to severity and duration) and a summary score were completed on the first and last days of the study period. The data are summarized in Tables 1.3 to 1.5.

The Brazelton Neonatal Behavior Assessment Scale (Brazelton 1973) was administered on the first and last days of the study period. These examinations were conducted by a trained graduate student or research assistant who was 'blind' to the infant's group assignment. The infant's performance was summarized according to the seven-cluster scoring criteria: habituation, orientation, motor behavior, range of state, regulation of state, autonomic stability, and abnormal reflexes (Lester & Brazelton 1982). In addition, the Neonatal Stress Behavior Scale (Eisen et al 1991) was completed based on stress behaviors observed during the examination.

## Results

Data analyses revealed that the groups were similar on all clinical measures at baseline (Table 1.3).

**Table 1.3** Means and standard deviations[1] for perinatal data (Study 2)

|  | Massage | | Control | | |
|---|---|---|---|---|---|
|  | Means | SD | Means | SD | p |
| Maternal age | 25.5 | 5.2 | 25.1 | 3.6 | NS |
| Parity | 4.1 | 2.6 | 3.7 | 1.2 | NS |
| Gestational age (weeks) | 29.7 | 1.9 | 30.8 | 2.1 | NS |
| Birth weight (g) | 1158.3 | 155.1 | 1265.4 | 206.6 | NS |
| Birth length (cm) | 36.8 | 2.9 | 38.8 | 3.4 | NS |
| Head circumference (cm) | 25.8 | 1.4 | 26.6 | 1.6 | NS |
| Ponderal index[2] | 2.4 | 0.5 | 2.2 | 0.4 | NS |
| Apgar |  |  |  |  |  |
| 1-min | 5.9 | 2.1 | 5.3 | 2.3 | NS |
| 5-min | 7.5 | 1.2 | 6.9 | 1.3 | NS |
| 10-min | 8.4 | 0.5 | 7.8 | 1.2 | NS |
| Obstetric complications[3] | 69.0 | 15.5 | 63.1 | 12.9 | NS |
| Postnatal complications[3] | 70.9 | 11.8 | 71.3 | 5.2 | NS |
| Newfoundland scale[4] | 7.1 | 3.4 | 7.2 | 4.1 | NS |
| Number of intensive care unit days | 20.3 | 14.5 | 16.2 | 8.3 | NS |
| Weight at study onset | 1458.0 | 118.7 | 1488.0 | 161.5 | NS |

[1] All comparisons were nonsignificant.
[2] Ponderal Index = birth weight/length$^3$ × 100.
[3] Higher score optimal.
[4] Lower score optimal.

**Table 1.4**  Means and standard deviations for clinical measures throughout the study period (Study 2)

|  | Massage | | Control | | |
|---|---|---|---|---|---|
|  | Means | SD | Means | SD | p |
| Respiration rate (breaths/min) | 54.8 | 2.3 | 54.0 | 3.1 | NS |
| Heart rate (beats/min) | 158.8 | 3.1 | 154.7 | 3.6 | 0.002 |
| Average temperature (°F) | 98.2 | 0.1 | 98.2 | 0.1 | NS |
| Frequency of stooling (1 day) | 1.6 | 0.5 | 1.3 | 0.6 | NS |
| Frequency of urination (1 day) | 8.2 | 0.4 | 8.1 | 0.5 | NS |
| Number of parent visits | 0.9 | 0.6 | 1.0 | 1.1 | NS |
| With touching | 0.8 | 1.7 | 1.0 | 1.1 | NS |
| With holding | 0.8 | 1.7 | 0.9 | 1.0 | NS |
| With feeding | 0.2 | 0.6 | 0.5 | 0.9 | NS |

Data analyses of the treatment effects suggested that both the massaged and control infants demonstrated fewer postnatal complications by the end of the study period (Table 1.5). However, the massaged infants showed significantly fewer complications than did the control infants at that time. Massaged infants also tended to show fewer postnatal complications on the Newfoundland Scale after the 10-day treatment period. Despite similar formula and caloric intake, the massaged infants averaged a 28% greater weight gain (mean = 33 g) than the control infants (mean = 26 g) over the treatment period (Table 1.6).

**Table 1.5**  Means and standard deviations for postnatal complications and stress symptoms (Study 2)

|  | Massage | | | | Control | | | | |
|---|---|---|---|---|---|---|---|---|---|
|  | Day 1 | | Day 10 | | Day 1 | | Day 10 | | |
|  | Means | SD | Means | SD | Means | SD | Means | SD | p[1] |
| Postnatal Complications Scale[2] | 68.6 | 7.7 | 95.7 | 9.1 | 71.3 | 5.2 | 78.9 | 3.6 | 0.005 |
| Newfoundland Scale[3] | 7.1 | 3.4 | 1.7 | 0.5 | 7.2 | 4.1 | 3.0 | 0.06 | NS |

[1] Significance for interaction effects.
[2] Higher score optimal.
[3] Lower score optimal.

**Table 1.6**   Means and standard deviations for intake and weight gain data (Study 2)

|  | Massage | | Control | | |
| --- | --- | --- | --- | --- | --- |
|  | Means | SD | Means | SD | p |
| Prestudy period | | | | | |
| Average weight gain | 24.3 | 9.4 | 32.5 | 21.2 | NS |
| Average feed type | 0.7 | 0.1 | 0.7 | 0.1 | NS |
| Average calories/kg | 153.1 | 27.5 | 144.1 | 22.6 | NS |
| Average fluid intake (mL/kg/day) | 200.1 | 31.8 | 199.4 | 31.2 | NS |
| During study period | | | | | |
| Average weight gain | 33.0 | 7.3 | 25.7 | 7.0 | 0.009 |
| Average feed type | 0.8 | 0.0 | 0.7 | 0.1 | NS |
| Average calories/kg | 120.1 | 10.8 | 113.1 | 12.7 | NS |
| Average fluid intake (mL/kg/day) | 154.8 | 9.8 | 153.7 | 10.7 | NS |
| Poststudy period | | | | | |
| Average weight gain | 31.5 | 16.0 | 29.6 | 10.5 | NS |
| Average feed type | 0.8 | 0.1 | 0.7 | 0.1 | NS |
| Average calories/kg | 248.3 | 42.1 | 227.4 | 48.6 | NS |
| Average fluid intake (mL/kg/day) | 314.3 | 48.2 | 307.1 | 55.3 | NS |

Analyses of the Brazelton Scale scores revealed that the massaged infants had better motor scores at the end of the 10-day study period, whereas the motor scores of the control infants remained the same. Also, the massaged infants tended to show improved orientation behaviors on the Brazelton Neonatal Behavior Assessment Scale by the end of the study period (Table 1.7). Furthermore, the massaged infants demonstrated significantly fewer stress behaviors by the last day, and the control infants remained the same across the treatment period.

**Table 1.7**   Means and standard deviations for the Brazelton clusters and performance (Study 2)

|  | Massage | | | | Control | | | | |
| --- | --- | --- | --- | --- | --- | --- | --- | --- | --- |
|  | Day 1 | | Day 10 | | Day 1 | | Day 10 | | |
|  | Means | SD | Means | SD | Means | SD | Means | SD | $p^1$ |
| Habituation | 5.7 | 1.2 | 6.0 | 1.0 | 6.6 | 0.5 | 6.4 | 0.8 | NS |
| Orientation | 3.9 | 2.2 | 4.9 | 1.5 | 3.2 | 2.5 | 3.2 | 2.4 | 0.06 |
| Motor maturity | 3.8 | 1.0 | 5.0 | 0.6 | 3.7 | 2.0 | 3.4 | 0.9 | 0.02 |
| Range of state | 3.6 | 1.1 | 4.1 | 0.9 | 2.7 | 1.2 | 3.5 | 1.1 | NS |
| Regulation of state | 4.6 | 1.6 | 5.9 | 1.0 | 3.0 | 1.2 | 4.8 | 1.2 | NS |
| Autonomic | 5.8 | 1.2 | 5.7 | 1.8 | 5.2 | 2.8 | 5.4 | 1.1 | NS |
| Reflexes[2] | 11.9 | 19.0 | 7.9 | 15.2 | 8.6 | 4.2 | 6.4 | 3.5 | NS |
| Stress behaviors[2] | 2.7 | 1.0 | 1.6 | 0.7 | 2.2 | 1.0 | 2.3 | 1.0 | 0.05 |

[1] Significance for interaction effects.
[2] Lower score optimal.

*Discussion*

These findings suggest that massage therapy can improve the clinical course of cocaine-exposed preterm infants. As cocaine-exposed newborns may experience more perinatal complications and neurological and behavioral abnormalities than nonexposed infants, massage therapy has important implications for intervention during the neonatal period. The massaged infants showed a 28% greater daily weight gain than control infants, although the groups did not differ on average intake (calories or volume). The massaged infants also experienced fewer postnatal complications and had more mature motor behaviors on the Brazelton examination as well as fewer stress behaviors and a tendency for better orientation performance after the 10-day massage treatment.

Although these findings are similar to those on preterm infants (Field et al 1986, Scafidi et al 1986, Scafidi et al 1990), this is the first investigation of massage effects on cocaine-exposed preterm infants. These findings, together with the increased weight gain and improved motor performance, suggest that massage contributed to the infants' wellbeing and made them appear more robust. This may facilitate early parent–infant interaction, which would in turn affect later development (Field et al 1984).

This investigation was the first to examine the effects of massage on cocaine-exposed preterm neonates. Findings of this study confirm previous findings on the benefits of massage and have important implications for intervention during the neonatal period. Because of the potential polydrug nature of this sample, the findings of the study might apply to drug-exposed infants in general.

## Study 3: HIV-exposed infants

Perinatal transmission is responsible for approximately 80% of all pediatric AIDS cases (Center for Disease Control, 1989). Pediatric AIDS and perinatal human immunodeficiency virus (HIV) infection are rapidly becoming the leading infectious causes of developmental delays (Armstrong, Seidel & Swales 1983; Belman et al 1988, Ultmann et al 1985). Further, AIDS is among the top ten causes of death in children aged 1 to 4 years (Kilbourne, Buehler & Rogers 1990). However, only approximately 22% to 39% of a sample of exposed infants might be expected to be diagnosed as HIV-positive themselves (Wolinsky et al 1992).

Very little research has been conducted on newborns exposed to HIV but not necessarily HIV-positive. In a study on Brazelton

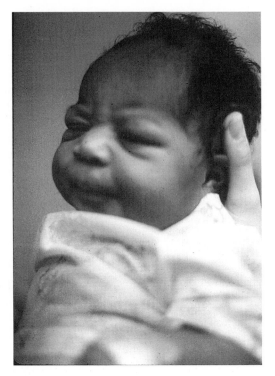

**Figure 1.4** HIV infant.

performance of HIV-exposed newborns, deficits were noted in the Brazelton performance of perinatal HIV-exposed versus non-exposed infants (Scafidi & Field 1996). However, in a study on older children, developmental delays were reported for the HIV-infected children but not for the noninfected but exposed children (Kletter et al 1989). Thus the data are mixed on children who are simply exposed. Nonetheless, because the exposed newborns showed inferior neonatal performance in the Scafidi & Field (1996) study and because at least 30% of a sample of exposed infants might be expected to be at risk for developmental delays due to infection, we investigated the effects of massage therapy with a sample of prenatally HIV-exposed newborns.

Again, because massage therapy has improved the behavior and development of preterm neonates, newborns of HIV-positive mothers were also expected to benefit. In a meta-analytic study, Ottenbacher and colleagues (Ottenbacher et al 1987) estimated that 72% of infants receiving tactile stimulation did better than nonstimulated control infants.

*Method*

**Sample** The sample was comprised of 28 singleton neonates (mean = 24 h) consecutively identified as HIV exposed and admitted to the study within 2 days after they were identified. The neonates were delivered vaginally and averaged 39 weeks gestation at birth and at the time of entry into the study. All infants remained in the nursery for monitoring for the 10-day duration of the study. The infants had no chromosomal aberrations, congenital heart malformations, gastrointestinal disturbances, perinatal complications, CNS dysfunctions, or infections such as meningitis and herpes encephalitis, and they were considered medically stable, free from ventilatory assistance, and were not receiving intravenous medications or feedings. A research associate randomly assigned (by a table of random numbers) the neonates to the treatment (massage therapy) or control groups. Both groups received the standard medical and nursing care and were being bottlefed without supplements in the neonatal intensive care unit. In addition to relatively high levels of ambient stimulation (sound and light) and a high nurse to infant ratio (1 to 2), volunteers held and fed the infants at 3-hour intervals. The average number of visits by parents was low (N = 4.8 for the 10-day period). The two groups did not differ on any birth parameters, and the women were all from a low education (mean = 10.5 years) and low socioeconomic background (mean = 4.5 on Hollingshead), and their ethnic distribution was 67% African-American and 33% Hispanic. Demographic and birth data are shown in Table 1.8.

**Procedures**

*Serological testing for human immunodeficiency virus (HIV-1) antibody.* All women were tested for human immunodeficiency virus. Maternal testing for HIV-1 antibody was performed using the ELISA method. A positive result was confirmed by the Western blot technique using nitrocellulose strips from Epitope. In the event that the mother's blood was positive, the infant's blood was also tested. Informed consent was obtained from the women to do HIV testing. The counselor obtaining consent explained the potential uses of the HIV test, its limitations, the meaning of test results, and an explanation of the procedures, including the voluntary nature of the testing, the right to withdraw consent at any time prior to HIV testing, and the confidential treatment of information identifying the subject.

*Urine toxicology and screens.* Routine urine toxicology screens were conducted on all mothers and infants eligible for this study. Enzyme immunoassays (EMIT) were used to measure cocaine metabolites (benzoylecgonine) and cannabinoids in maternal urine. Maternal specimens were also assayed for five additional substances (opiates, amphetamines, barbiturates, benzodiazepines, and phycyclidine). Due to the difficulty in obtaining adequate volumes of urine, the infants' samples were limited to three assays: cocaine metabolites, cannabinoids, and opiates. If maternal urine was not obtained, the five assays listed for maternal urine were performed on the infant sample. Mothers and infants had negative urine toxicologies.

*Obstetric and postnatal data.* Obstetric complications were quantified using the Obstetric Complications Scale (Littman & Parmelee 1978). Perinatal complications were quantified using the Perinatal Risk Index (Scheiner & Sexton 1991). This 14-item scale weights complications on a four-point scale according to severity and duration. Items include: Apgar scores, EEG, presence of seizures, intracranial hemorrhage, presence of hydrocephalus, head ultrasound, weight for gestational age (2 items), dysmorphic features, ventilation, hematocrit, meningitis, and head growth (2 items).

*Neonatal Behavior Assessment Scale–Kansas Supplements.* The Brazelton Neonatal Behavior Assessment Scale (Brazelton 1973) was administered to each infant midway between feedings in a sleep state prior to and following the 10-day stimulation period. The infant's performance was summarized according to seven factors: habituation, orientation, motor behavior, range of state, regulation of state, autonomic stability and abnormal reflexes (Lester et al 1982). In addition, excitability and depression were scored as suggested using a scoring system designed by Lester and Tronick (unpublished). Finally, the infants' stressful responses to Brazelton scale items were scored according to a system designed by Eisen and colleagues (Eisen et al 1991). Examiners blind to group membership conducted these assessments in a quiet small closet-like room adjacent to the nursery.

*Massage therapy.* The same massage that was used in our previous studies was provided to the massage therapy group infants for three 15-minute periods during 3 consecutive hours each day for a 10-day period (Monday–Friday) (Field et al 1986). Massage therapy was not provided on the intervening weekend. The first stimulation session was begun approximately 30 minutes following the noon feeding, the second session began approximately 45 minutes after completion of the first session, and the third session began approximately 45 minutes after completion of the second session. The 15-minute stimulation session was comprised of three standardized 5-minute phases.

The first and third phases were tactile, and the middle phase was kinesthetic stimulation just as in Study 1 (this chapter).

## Results

Data analyses suggested that the massage therapy and control groups were initially equivalent at the start of the study (Table 1.9). On the Brazelton Scale the massage therapy group had more optimal score changes on several clusters. These included habituation, motor, range of state and autonomic stability scores. The massage therapy group also received better scores on excitability and stress behaviors. Finally, the massage therapy group averaged a significantly greater increase in weight gain.

## Discussion

The results of this study are perhaps not surprising given the superior performance on the Brazelton Neonatal Behavior Scale and greater weight gain noted following 2 weeks of massage therapy in the previous studies already described (Field et al 1986, Kuhn et al 1991, Scafidi et al 1990). However, even though the infants in the study were lower in gestational age and birth weight than normal, which is not surprising for infants with HIV, they had longer gestation and larger birth weight than the infants of the previous massage studies. Therefore, the significant weight gain following extra stimulation would be more surprising.

**Table 1.8**  Means (and standard deviations in parentheses) for demographic and birth measures (Study 3)

| Variable | Massage | Control |
|---|---|---|
| Mother's SES | 4.4   (0.8) | 4.6   (0.9) |
| Mother's education | 10.6   (1.1) | 10.4   (1.3) |
| Mother's age | 26.3   (3.2) | 27.7   (4.3) |
| Mother's parity | 3.4   (0.2) | 3.4   (0.3) |
| OCS | 88.6   (19.4) | 93.1   (18.9) |
| Gestational age (weeks) | 38.6   (1.9) | 38.9   (1.1) |
| Birth weight (g) | 3164.2   (663) | 2881.4   (619) |
| Length (cm) | 49.5   (6.2) | 48.1   (5.9) |
| Ponderal Index[1] | 2.5   (0.3) | 2.5   (0.5) |
| Head circumference | 33.1   (3.8) | 33.4   (3.1) |
| APGAR (1 min) | 7.4   (0.6) | 7.6   (0.4) |
| APGAR (5 min) | 8.7   (0.7) | 8.9   (0.6) |
| Postnatal factors | 9.4   (17.8) | 9.2   (15.3) |

[1] This Ponderal Index (just above the 10th percentile) suggests some intrauterine growth deprivation.

**Table 1.9** Means (and standard deviations in parentheses) for Brazelton Neonatal Behavior Assessment Scale scores and daily weight gain (Study 3)

| Brazelton score | Massage | | Control | | $p^5$ |
|---|---|---|---|---|---|
| | Day 1 | Day 10 | Day 1 | Day 10 | |
| Habituation[1] | 6.9[4] | 6.8 | 6.2 | 4.6 | 0.01 |
| | (0.6)$_a$ | (0.4)$_a$ | (0.5)$_a$ | (0.5)$_b$ | |
| Orientation[1] | 3.6 | 4.5 | 3.8 | 4.4 | NS |
| | (0.2)$_a$ | (0.3)$_a$ | (0.4)$_a$ | (0.5)$_a$ | |
| Motor[1] | 4.3 | 5.2 | 3.8 | 4.5 | 0.001 |
| | (0.5)$_a$ | (0.5)$_b$ | (0.4)$_a$ | (0.4)$_a$ | |
| Range of state[1] | 3.5 | 4.3 | 3.2 | 3.6 | 0.05 |
| | (0.3)$_a$ | (0.4)$_b$ | (0.5)$_a$ | (0.3)$_a$ | |
| Regulation of state[1] | 4.7 | 4.0 | 5.4 | 4.5 | NS |
| | (0.4)$_a$ | (0.6)$_a$ | (0.6)$_a$ | (0.7)$_a$ | |
| Autonomic stability[1] | 5.8 | 6.2 | 6.0 | 5.0 | 0.003 |
| | (0.5)$_a$ | (0.7)$_b$ | (0.8)$_a$ | (0.5)$_a$ | |
| Reflexes[2] | 3.3 | 2.2 | 3.2 | 2.7 | NS |
| | (0.2)$_a$ | (0.3)$_a$ | (0.4)$_a$ | (0.2)$_a$ | |
| Excitability[2] | 2.5 | 1.5 | 1.8 | 3.2 | 0.01 |
| | (0.2)$_a$ | (0.4)$_b$ | (0.3)$_b$ | (0.4)$_a$ | |
| Depression[2] | 3.5 | 3.0 | 4.8 | 2.9 | NS |
| | (0.5)$_a$ | (0.4)$_a$ | (0.5)$_a$ | (0.4)$_a$ | |
| Stress behaviors[2] | 2.4 | 1.8 | 1.8 | 3.6 | 0.004 |
| | (0.2)$_a$ | (0.2)$_b$ | (0.4)$_b$ | (0.5)$_a$ | |
| Daily weight gain[3] | 22.5 | 33.4 | 20.2 | 26.3 | 0.01 |
| | (2.4)$_a$ | (4.3)$_b$ | (3.7)$_a$ | (3.9)$_a$ | |

[1] Higher score is optimal.
[2] Lower score is optimal.
[3] Day 1 means the 1st day of the study, although it was on average the 3rd day of life for the infants.
[4] Different subscript letters indicate significant differences between columns.
[5] Using the more conservative Bonferroni correction factor the range of state factor would not be significant.

Many of the Brazelton Neonatal Behavior Scale score differences were accounted for by the massage therapy group improving and by the control group remaining the same or declining. These trends are very different than those noted in the earlier massage therapy studies on massaged preterm infants who simply improved more than the control group preemies. The preterm control groups did not stay the same or decline but improved in their performance, as would be expected with development. Exposure to HIV may contribute to developing delays and failure-to-thrive as early as the newborn period in the absence of compensatory treatment provided by extra stimulation. It is also possible that these effects resulted from other risk conditions such as maternal drug use that could not be detected by our urine screens or by intrauterine growth deprivation. Nonetheless, the surprising finding was the unusual number of inferior scores received by the control infants with HIV on several Brazelton Scale dimensions, suggesting a generalized, pervasive influence of HIV on newborn behaviors. The early appearance of delay and failure to thrive in the control group is somewhat surprising given that supposedly only 22% to 39% of these infants reputedly remain HIV positive (Blanche et al 1989, Johnson et al 1989, Peckham et al 1990). However, the perinatal exposure could contribute even to developing atrophy of the cerebral cortex, calcification of the basal ganglia, and deterioration of white matter, even in a small subgroup, and negatively affect the group comparisons (Barnes 1986, Belman 1990, Curless 1989).

On the positive side, deterioration in HIV-exposed newborns apparently can be attenuated by the use of massage therapy. The underlying mechanisms linking stimulation to weight gain, and stimulation to improved performance, are not clear. The weight gain may relate to increased vagal activity following massage, which in turn facilitates the release of food absorption hormones such as insulin noted in our study on preemies exposed to cocaine (Scafidi et al 1996). Better performance on the Brazelton could also relate to increased vagal activity, as better performing infants typically have higher vagal activity (Porges 1985).

In a more recent study on HIV-exposed infants, the mothers of the infants were used as the massage therapists (Fig. 1.5). The mothers' treatment compliance rates were very high, perhaps because of the guilt they expressed for having possibly transmitted HIV to their infants and their own high anxiety levels (Scafidi & Field 1996). Teaching parents to massage their infants often lowers their anxiety levels related to their feeling helpless about their infant's or their child's condition. Helping with their children's treatment might be expected to decrease their anxiety levels and make them feel that they were contributing to the treatment. Also, massages can be given to children on a daily basis, as they are economically feasible when the parents are used as therapists. In the HIV-exposed infants, the massaged infants' weight gain was significantly greater and they showed significantly fewer stress behaviors than the nonmassaged control infants.

# NORMAL INFANTS
## Study 4: Normal infants also benefit from massage therapy

Because all three groups of high-risk infants had been helped by the massage therapy, we wondered if normal or nonrisk infants

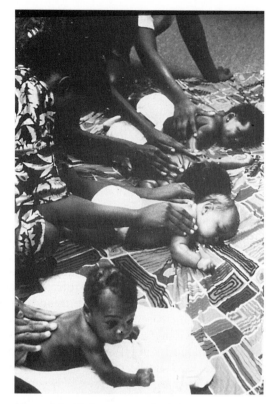

**Figure 1.5** Mothers massaging infants.

might also benefit. Although research on infant massage is limited, therapists have suggested (Auckett 1981) that massage:

1. reduces stress responses to painful procedures, such as inoculations
2. reduces pain associated with teething, constipation and colic
3. helps induce sleep
4. makes parents (who are typically the massage therapists) 'feel good' while they are massaging their infants
5. facilitates parent–infant bonding and the development of warm, positive relationships.

Although the massage therapy benefits for high-risk preterm infants are clear, the benefits of massage for full-term infants had not been explored. Full-term infants were expected to benefit as well, and particularly full-term infants born to high-risk mothers such as depressed mothers. Several studies have documented less positive affect in infants of depressed mothers (Cohn et al 1986,

Field 1984); and more recently, growth delays and inferior performance on developmental assessments have been noted in infants of depressed mothers (Field 1992). Massaging these infants was expected to improve their affect and growth, as it did with preterm infants (Field et al 1986). Based upon previous research we expected to find that massaging these infants would have the following effects:

• greater daily weight gain
• more organized sleep/wake behaviors
• less fussiness and more positive affect
• lower cortisol levels and higher norepinephrine levels.

## Method

**Sample** The sample was comprised of 40 full-term 1- to 3-month-old infants born to adolescent depressed mothers. The infants were recruited at birth and attended our daycare nursery from birth and during the time they participated in the study. The infants were born full-term (mean gestational age = 39.4 weeks, range = 37–41), were normal birth weight (mean = 3483 g, range = 3120–3610), and had normal Apgar scores (mean = 9.1, range = 6–10; see Table 1.10). Their mothers were categorized as low SES (mean = 4.2, range = 3.1–5.0) on the Hollingshead Index, were single parents, were adolescents (mean age = 17.3 years, range = 14–19) and were primary caregivers on public assistance; 65% were African American, 35% were Hispanic. The infants were randomly assigned to a massage therapy group or a rocking control group. The two groups did not differ on any of the maternal demographic characteristics (see Table 1.10) based on chi-square analysis of their ethnic distribution and $t$ tests of their socioeconomic status (SES). In addition, the groups did not differ on infant birth characteristics based on $t$ tests, nor on sex distribution based on chi-square analysis.

The mothers were classified depressed because they were diagnosed dysthymic on the Diagnostic Interview Schedule (DIS; Costello, Edelbrock, & Costello 1985) and had Beck Depression Inventory scores greater than 16 (mean = 28.1) (Beck et al 1961).

**Diagnostic Interview Schedule (DIS)** The DIS is a standardized diagnostic interview that addresses specific symptoms as well as their chronology, duration, and associated impairments. The interview has a step structure that minimizes interviewing time. The questions are precoded 0–1–2, corresponding to 'no,' 'somewhat or sometimes,' and 'yes.' Reliability and validity of the DIS have been found to be as good or better than other structured diagnostic interviews (Costello et al 1985). The interviews for this

**Table 1.10**  Demographic and birth characteristics[1] (Study 4)

|  | Group | | |
|  | Massage therapy | Rocking | p |
| --- | --- | --- | --- |
| Demographic variables | | | |
| Ethnicity | | | |
| Black (%)[2] | 66 | 64 | NS |
| Hispanic (%)[2] | 34 | 36 | NS |
| SES[3] | 4.1  (1.3) | 4.3  (1.5) | NS |
| Birth characteristics[3] | | | |
| Gestational age (weeks) | 39.2  (2.2) | 39.6  (2.1) | NS |
| Birth weight (g) | 3477.1  (123.2) | 3489.2  (116.0) | NS |
| Apgar score | 9.0  (1.1) | 9.1  (1.2) | NS |

[1] Values are means with standard deviations in parentheses.
[2] Chi-square analyses were used for group comparisons on this variable.
[3] $t$ tests were performed to compare groups on this variable.

study were conducted by one interviewer who had received training at a national DIS training workshop. For this study, only the Affective Disorder Module was used to assess depression.

The initial diagnosis was made following the infant's delivery. Another diagnosis was made at the beginning of the study. If a mother was no longer diagnosed depressed, she was not recruited for the study. Only 4% of the mothers were no longer depressed by the time of the study.

During the study the infants were cared for during the day by teachers at our nursery school. The infants were bottle-fed by nursery caregivers except when the mothers visited. The mothers routinely touched, held, and fed their infants, and this was recorded (presence/absence of each of the behaviors) by the teachers on a daily basis. The groups did not differ based on the teachers' daily record of the amount of time the mothers visited, touched, held, and fed their infants. In addition,the mothers were unaware of which therapy their infants were receiving (massage or rocking) and were unaware of the intent of the study, as were the teachers.

**Procedures**

*Massage therapy.* The massage therapy infants (N = 20) were provided a 15-minute massage midway between morning feedings 2 days per week for a 6-week period. The infant was placed in a supine position on a comfortable mat in a quiet area of the nursery. The massage therapy was administered by a researcher who was trained in the procedure. The therapist placed a small amount of mineral baby oil on the palms of her warm hands and placed her hands on the infant's chest. She then worked on the following six regions of the infant's body:

1. *face*:
   (a) firm strokes with the flats of the fingers along both sides of the face and across the forehead
   (b) circular strokes over the temples and the hinge of the jaw
   (c) strokes with the flats of the fingers over the nose, cheeks, jaw and chin
2. *chest*:
   (a) strokes along both sides of the chest with the flats of the fingers, going from the middle outward
   (b) cross strokes from the center of the chest and over the shoulders
   (c) strokes on both sides of the chest simultaneously with flats of the hands over the chest to the shoulders.
3. *stomach*:
   (a) hand-over-hand motion in a paddlewheel fashion going from higher to lower region
   (b) circular motion with fingers in a clockwise direction starting at the appendix
4. *legs/feet*:
   (a) long strokes from hip to foot
   (b) squeezing and twisting in a wringing motion from foot to hip
   (c) long milking stokes toward the heart from foot to hip
   (d) long strokes toward the heart from foot to hip
5. *arms*:
   (a) long strokes from shoulder to hand
   (b) squeezing and twisting in a wringing motion from hand to shoulder
   (c) long milking strokes toward the heart from hand to shoulder
   (d) long strokes toward the heart from hand to shoulder
6. *back* (the infant was placed in a prone position):
   (a) hand over hand motion in a paddlewheel fashion from upper back to buttocks with flats of the hands contoured to the shape of the back
   (b) hands from side to side across the infant's back, including sides
   (c) circular motion with fingertips, from head to buttocks over the long muscles next to the spine (not directly rubbing the spine)
   (d) simultaneous strokes over both sides of the back from the middle to the sides
   (e) with finger tips rub and knead the shoulder muscles
   (f) with finger tips rub the neck
   (g) strokes along length of the back
   (h) strokes from the head to the feet.

*Rocking group.* Rocking was used both as an attention (one-on-one) control and a physical contact control for the massage therapy group. It was also used as a relatively conservative test for massage therapy effects, inasmuch as rocking itself reduces fussiness and induces sleep – effects we also expected for the massage therapy. The rocking group (N = 20 infants) was scheduled for rocking sessions at the same time of day as the massage group (15 minutes on 2 days per days per week over 6 weeks for 12 sessions). During this condition, the infant was held in a cradled position by the researcher and rocked in a rocking chair. This control condition was employed to ensure that any changes noted in behavior/physiology were not related simply to changes in activity or to the physical presence/attention provided by the researcher.

**Immediate-effects measures (during and after treatment sessions on first and last days)**

*Sleep/wake/behavior.* To determine the immediate effects of the therapies on sleep/wake behavior, the infants were observed by a researcher during and for 15 minutes after the massage and rocking sessions on the first and last days of the study period. The observer recorded the infant's predominant state and various behaviors using a time-sampling unit methodology with 10 s recording intervals. An adaptation of Thoman's (Thoman et al 1981) system of sleep recording was used. The sleep state criteria were as follows:

1. quiet sleep (no REM) – the infant's eyes are closed and still, and there is no motor activity other than an occasional startle, rhythmic mouthing, or a slight limb movement
2. active sleep (without REM) – the infant's eyes are closed and still; motor activity is present
3. REM sleep – the infant's eyes are closed, although they may open briefly; rapid eye movements can be detected through closed eyelids, and motor activity may or may not be present
4. drowsy – the infant's eyes may be opening and closing but have a dull, glazed appearance; motor activity is minimal
5. inactive alert – the infant is relatively inactive, although there may be occasional limb movements; the eyes are wide open and bright and shiny
6. active awake – the infant's eyes are open and there is motor activity
7. crying – the infant's eyes can be open or closed, and motor activity is present, as are agitated vocalizations.

In addition to coding behavioral states, the observer also recorded: (a) single-limb movements; (b) multiple-limb movements; (c) gross body movements; (d) head turning; (e) facial grimaces; (f) startles; (g) mouthing; (h) smiles; and (i) clenched fists.

Totals for time-sample units were converted to the percentage of observation time for which different states and behaviors occurred, for the purposes of data analysis. To ensure reliability of the coding, the observer was first trained to a criterion of 90% reliability (number of agreements/number of agreements plus disagreements) prior to the onset of the study. Interobserver reliability was then determined during the course of the study by the simultaneous observation and coding of 10 randomly selected sleep observations which were videotaped. The coding was done simultaneously to ensure that the start and end points were synchronized. The coders used laptop computers and were separated by a post so they could not observe each other's coding. The reliability coefficients were calculated by dividing the number of agreements (same behaviors coded for a given time-sampling unit by both observers) by the number of agreements and disagreements. The reliability coefficients averaged 0.84.

*Salivary cortisol.* Saliva samples were obtained immediately before and 20 minutes after the massage and rocking sessions (held between the morning feeding sessions on the first and last days of the study). They were assayed to determine any changes in cortisol levels as a general index of stress. Due to the 20-minute lag between plasma and salivary cortisol levels, saliva samples reflected stress states at 20 minutes prior to the session and immediately following the session. The saliva samples were frozen and later assayed for cortisol levels at Duke University.

**Longer-term measures (first day/last day)**

*Weight and formula intake data.* Volume of daytime formula intake was recorded daily by the infant caregivers. The mothers also recorded the number of night-time bottle feedings. In addition, the infants were weighed daily immediately prior to the early morning feeding.

*Temperament rating.* On the first and last days of the treatment period, the Colorado Child Temperament Inventory (CCTI) (Rowe & Plomin 1977) was completed by the infants' nursery school teachers who are masters degree teachers and who received reliability training to the 0.90 level on the CCTI. Inter-rater reliability between teachers and psychology graduate students based on 30% of the sample yielded kappa coefficients ranging from 0.73 to 0.87 (mean = 0.82). This scale is comprised of 30 Likert-type (strongly disagree to strongly agree) statements such as 'Infant tends to be shy' and 'Infant is always on the go'. This scale yields six factors, the same in this sample as in the normative sample

(Rowe & Plomin 1977): emotionality, activity, sociability, soothability, persistence and food adaptation. Test–retest reliability is
good, r = 0.89, and validity has been assessed in relation to interaction ratings made by independent observers which yielded
high correlations ranging from 0.83 to 0.91 (Field 1992).

*Urine assays.* First morning urine samples were collected on the
first and last days of the study. The urine samples were frozen
and sent to Duke University for assays. Urine assays of norepinephrine, epinephrine, and serotonin (5H1AA) were conducted
by high-pressure liquid chromatography with electrochemical
detection; cortisol was determined by radioimmune assay; and
creatinine was assayed calorimetrically (Kuhn et al 1991).

## Results

As can be seen in Table 1.11, the massage therapy infants were
in a different state during the sessions than the rocking group.
The massage therapy infants spent more time in inactive alert and
active awake states (also moving more) and less time in drowsy
and quiet sleep states. In addition, their crying and salivary cortisol
levels decreased – unlike the rocking group infants, whose crying
and cortisol levels remained the same. The rocked infants spent
less time in an active awake state during the rocking session, but
were awake after the rocking session, suggesting that massage
may be more effective than rocking for inducing sleep.

As can be seen in Table 1.12, several long-term differences were
noted for the massage group infants across the course of the
study – as opposed to the rocking group infants, who did not
change. The massage therapy infants:

- gained weight, although no change occurred in formula intake
- improved on temperament dimensions, including
  emotionality, sociability, and soothability
- experienced decreases in urinary catecholamine and cortisol
  levels and increased serotonin levels.

## Discussion

The greater alertness the infants experienced during massage
therapy is consistent with data on adults showing EEG changes
that conform to a pattern of alertness, namely decreased alpha and
beta waves (Field, Ironson et al 1996). Improved performance on
math tasks (less time required and fewer errors) accompanied the
EEG pattern of alertness in the same adults receiving massage.
The increased alertness data are also consistent with increased

**Table 1.11**  Means (and SDs) for sleep/wake behaviors during and after sessions for massage therapy and rocking groups[1] (Study 4)

|  | Massage therapy | | Rocking | |  |
| --- | --- | --- | --- | --- | --- |
| Variables | During | After | During | After | p |
| Sleep/wake behaviors |  |  |  |  |  |
| Quiet sleep | 4.3 $(2.0)_a$ | 48.1 $(26.0)_b$ | 45.9 $(21.0)_b$ | 41.8 $(18.0)_b$ | 0.001 |
| Active sleep | 0.0 $(0.0)_a$ | 4.8 $(2.0)_a$ | 0.0 $(0.0)_a$ | 0.0 $(0.0)_a$ | NS |
| Rem sleep | 0.0 $(0.0)_a$ | 2.9 $(2.0)_a$ | 3.1 $(2.0)_a$ | 0.0 $(0.0)_a$ | NS |
| Drowsy | 0.8 $(0.0)_a$ | 5.3 $(3.0)_b$ | 4.3 $(3.0)_b$ | 7.3 $(4.0)_b$ | 0.05 |
| Inactive alert | 35.6 $(16.0)_a$ | 23.6 $(14.0)_b$ | 16.7 $(11.0)_{bc}$ | 10.9 $(6.0)_c$ | 0.05 |
| Active awake | 46.2 $(26.0)_a$ | 14.3 $(9.0)_b$ | 21.7 $(11.0)_c$ | 29.3 $(14.0)_c$ | 0.001 |
| Crying | 14.4 $(12.0)_a$ | 2.5 $(2.0)_b$ | 8.3 $(6.0)_a$ | 10.7 $(9.0)_a$ | 0.001 |
| Movement | 87.7 $(39.0)_a$ | 44.1 $(21.0)_b$ | 45.3 $(23.0)_b$ | 56.7 $(27.0)_b$ | 0.001 |
| Saliva cortisol[2] | 2.1 $(1.0)_a$ | 1.4 $(1.0)_b$ | 1.9 $(1.0)_{ab}$ | 1.6 $(1.0)_b$ | 0.05 |

[1] Different subscript letters denote significant differences.
[2] Saliva cortisol values taken before and after session.

**Table 1.12**  Means (and SDs) for variables measured at beginning and end of study period for massage therapy and rocking group infants[1] (Study 4)

|  | Massage therapy | | Rocking | |  |
| --- | --- | --- | --- | --- | --- |
| Variables | Day 1 | Day 12 | Day 1 | Day 12 | p |
| Weight (lb) | 14.7 $(3.0)_a$ | 16.3 $(3.0)_b$ | 14.9 $(3.0)_a$ | 15.4 $(3.0)_a$ | 0.001 |
| Formula intake | 7.0 $(3.0)_a$ | 8.4 $(3.0)_a$ | 8.0 $(3.0)_a$ | 10.8 $(4.0)_a$ | NS |
| Temperament |  |  |  |  |  |
| Emotionality[2] | 13.7 $(3.0)_a$ | 12.2 $(4.0)_b$ | 13.6 $(5.0)_a$ | 13.0 $(5.0)_a$ | 0.05 |
| Activity | 17.9 $(6.0)_a$ | 17.6 $(4.0)_a$ | 16.4 $(4.0)_a$ | 16.0 $(5.0)_a$ | NS |
| Sociability[3] | 18.5 $(3.0)_a$ | 19.9 $(4.0)_b$ | 19.1 $(5.0)_b$ | 18.4 $(4.0)_a$ | 0.05 |
| Soothability[3] | 16.5 $(4.0)_a$ | 18.5 $(4.0)_b$ | 15.8 $(5.0)_a$ | 15.6 $(5.0)_a$ | 0.05 |
| Persistence | 16.5 $(3.0)_a$ | 16.7 $(4.0)_a$ | 16.1 $(4.0)_a$ | 16.8 $(4.0)_a$ | NS |
| Food adaptation | 14.1 $(4.0)_a$ | 13.4 $(4.0)_a$ | 14.1 $(6.0)_a$ | 13.9 $(4.0)_b$ | NS |
| Biochemical measures[4] |  |  |  |  |  |
| Norepinephrine[2] | 245.3 $(139.0)_a$ | 119.7 $(77.0)_b$ | 195.0 $(94.0)_a$ | 180.0 $(89.0)_a$ | 0.05 |
| Epinephrine[2] | 21.5 $(14.0)_a$ | 10.6 $(6.0)_b$ | 16.0 $(10.0)_a$ | 23.6 $(15.0)_a$ | 0.05 |
| Serotonin (5H1AA)[3] | 944.9 $(581.0)_a$ | 1427.9 $(779.0)_b$ | 1001.5 $(492.0)_a$ | 1132.4 $(517.0)_a$ | 0.05 |
| Cortisol (urine)[2] | 1382.9 $(717.0)_a$ | 656.4 $(340.0)_b$ | 1225.4 $(639.0)_a$ | 1016.8 $(523.0)_a$ | 0.05 |

[1] Different subscript letters denote significant differences.
[2] Lower value is optimal.
[3] Higher value is optimal.
[4] Biochemical measures expressed as ng/g creatinine.

attentiveness accompanying increased vagal activity during massage therapy (Field & Schanberg 1990).

Rocking, in contrast, contributed to drowsiness and quiet sleep states during the rocking, but the greater arousal after the rocking was consistent with anecdotal reports from parents that rocking cessation often awakens the infant. These data, combined with the decreases noted in crying and salivary cortisol levels of the massaged versus the rocked infants, suggest that massage may be more effective than rocking for inducing sleep.

The longer-term gains made by the massaged versus the rocked infants are perhaps more surprising. Although several studies have reported that preterm infants gained more weight following massage (Field et al 1986, Ottenbacher et al 1987, Scafidi et al 1990), the baseline weights of the full-term infants in this study were higher. Thus, the massage might not be expected to increase their weight. They did, however, show greater weight gain, even though a difference of 1.1 lb might not be considered clinically significant. Nonetheless, the data suggest that because infants of chronically depressed mothers are noted to show growth delays by 1 year (Field 1992) and because massage is an easy technique for mothers to learn, this may be an effective measure for sustaining weight gain.

Improved ratings on emotionality and sociability temperament dimensions suggest that the massage enhanced the infants' responsivity to social stimulation. Increased soothability and decreased stress levels, as suggested by lower cortisol and catecholamine levels, may have also contributed to the infants' enhanced responsivity.

In summary, these data suggest that massage therapy may enhance the behavior and development of infants of depressed mothers. The infants were first more alert and then showed less stress, and their sleep was enhanced. Over the treatment period, they gained more weight, appeared less stressed (lower cortisol and catecholamines), and were more soothable and more sociable. These changes suggest that this therapy may be an effective way for depressed mothers to enhance their infants' development. Further research will be required to determine the underlying mechanisms for these massage therapy effects.

## POTENTIAL UNDERLYING MECHANISMS

The research by Schanberg and colleagues presented earlier plus the work of Uvnas-Moberg in Sweden suggested to us the potential underlying mechanism for the relationship between massage therapy and weight gain. Uvnas-Moberg and her colleagues (1987) reported that stimulating the inside of the mouth of the newborn (and the breast of the mother) led to the increased release of gastrointestinal food absorption hormones, including gastrin and insulin. We expected that stimulating the entire body, as in massage therapy, would lead to even higher levels of food absorption hormones mediated by vagal activity. Vagal activity did increase during massage therapy in one of our studies (Field & Schanberg 1990), and the vegetative branch of the vagus is known to stimulate the release of food absorption hormones, including insulin and gastrin. As already mentioned, assays of (heelstick) blood samples of preterm cocaine-exposed infants yielded significantly elevated insulin levels in those infants who were massaged (Scafidi et al 1996). Even though the branch of the vagus that slows down the heart and the branch that stimulates the release of food absorption hormones are different, vagal activity and the release of food absorption hormones appear to be related.

The superior habituation performance noted at the neonatal period in our preterm infant studies and superior performance on the Bayley mental scale at 1 year may derive from enhanced hippocampal development. Meaney and his colleagues (1990) noted increased glucocorticoids, decreased dendritic arborization in the hippocampal region, and inferior maze performance, suggesting impaired memory function in aging rats that had been deprived of tactile stimulation as rat pups. Similarly, the more elaborate dendritic arborization in the MRIs of the hippocampal region of massaged preterm neonates expected by Modi and colleagues (Modi & Glover 1996) suggests that massage therapy enhances brain development.

In a recent study we attempted to determine which newborns would benefit the most from massage therapy (Scafidi et al 1996). Ninety-three preterm infants (mean gestational age = 30 weeks; mean birth weight = 1204 g; mean ICU duration = 15 days) were randomly assigned to a massage therapy group or a control group once they were considered medically stable. The treatment group ($N = 50$) received three daily 15-minute massages for 10 days. The massage therapy infants gained significantly more weight per day (32 vs 29 g) than did the control infants. Treatment and control groups were divided into high and low weight gainers based on the average weight gain for the control group. Seventy percent of the massage therapy infants were classified as high weight gainers, whereas only 40% of the control infants were classified as high weight gainers. Discriminant function analysis determining the characteristics that distinguished the high from the low weight gainers suggested that the control infants who, before the study, consumed more calories and spent less time in intermediate care gained more weight. In contrast, for the massage therapy group, the pattern of greater caloric intake and more days in intermediate care before the study period, along with a higher number of obstetric complications, differentiated the high from the low weight gainers, suggesting that the infants who had experienced more complications before the study benefitted more from the massage therapy. These variables can be used to suggest infants who would benefit most from future massage therapy programs.

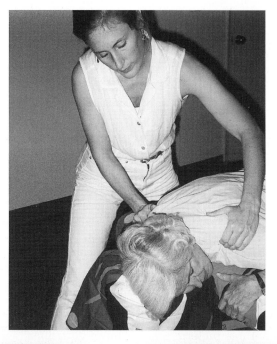

a

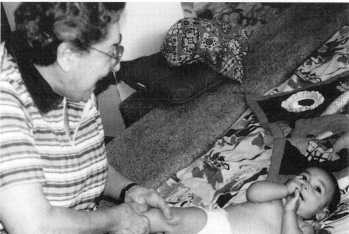

b

**Figure 1.6**  (a) 'Grandparent' volunteer being massaged. (b) 'Grandparent' volunteer massaging infant.

## Study 5: 'Grandparent' volunteers as therapists

Given the success of massage therapy for infants, it is possible that it will be used more frequently in the future. However, it will first be necessary to find a cost-effective way to administer massage therapy. We expected that one inexpensive source of therapists would be elder retired volunteers who provide various kinds of caregiving. We also expected that the elder volunteers would benefit from the human contact they received as they massage infants. Similar benefits have been observed in other forms of therapy. Pet therapy, for example, has had positive effects on aging people who are deprived of physical contact (Grossberg & Alf 1985, Vormbrock & Grossberg 1988). Siegel (1990) found that elderly individuals who owned pets reported fewer doctor contacts over a 1 year period than those who did not own pets. Research to date had only focused on the effects of receiving massage. Nothing was known about the effects on the person giving the massage.

Elder volunteers at hospitals and health care facilities seemed to be a good source for several reasons:

1. They volunteer their time and their services at no cost.
2. They are generally retired individuals who have the extra time needed to devote special attention to the care of others.
3. Research shows that some elderly people are prone to feelings of loneliness, depression, and decreased immune functioning.

Because massage is noted to decrease depression and enhance immune function (see later chapters), the elder retired volunteers may benefit themselves from the extra touch they receive from providing massage (Hendrie & Crosset 1990, McCullough 1991, Ruegg, Zisook & Swerdlow 1988). For these reasons, this group was considered ideal for examining the effects of giving massages.

The aim of this exploratory study was to examine the therapeutic effects of elder retired volunteers giving massages. We predicted that the volunteers would have increased social contacts, fewer depressive symptoms, improved sleep and eating patterns, and enhanced self-esteem.

*Method*

**Participants** The sample was comprised of ten elder volunteers (eight females; mean age = 70.0). The elder volunteers were Caucasian ($N = 6$) or Hispanic ($N = 4$), middle SES (3.1 on the Hollingshead Index for socioeconomic status) and averaged 15 years education. Half were married and half saw other family members only infrequently (monthly or holidays only). None of the volunteers was on medications and none of them was experiencing any chronic medical conditions. Only four of the volunteers had previously received a massage. This information suggested that receiving massage was a novel experience for this sample.

The ten elder volunteers massaged the ten healthy, full-term 1–3-month-old infants at the infants' daycare center three times a week for 3 weeks, and they received massage themselves at a nearby clinic three times a week for 3 weeks. The frequency and duration of the massage period was based on previous studies showing that this was an adequate treatment time to demonstrate effects in this size sample (Field et al 1992). The order of giving and receiving massages was counterbalanced. That is, one-half of the volunteers gave massage for the first 3 weeks and then received massage for 3 weeks, and the other half received massage for the first 3 weeks and then gave massage for the second 3 weeks. Thus, the volunteers served as their own controls.

**Giving massage** For the giving massage condition, Swedish massage techniques were taught to the elder retired volunteers by a trained research assistant. The volunteers massaged their assigned infant three times a week for 3 weeks for a total of nine massages. The more complex massage used in Study 4 was used here because these infants were slightly older and thus would prefer a more varied massage. Each massage lasted 15 minutes (see Study 4).

**Receiving massage** The elder volunteers received a 30-minute massage by a trained therapist three times a week for 3 weeks, for a total of nine massages. Their massage also consisted of Swedish massage techniques and focused on the face, neck, shoulders, arms, legs, back and feet but was twice as long as the infants' massage because at least twice the body surface needed to be massaged in the elder volunteers versus the infants. For the first 15 minutes the massage was performed in the face-up position and for the last 15 minutes it was administered face-down. The massage began with lengthening and stretching of the neck and spine, followed by stroking of the forehead and face. This was followed by depression of the shoulders and the application of pressure to the tender points. The arms and legs were stretched and the arms were lifted and moved in a slow circular motion. Short, smooth strokes were used to massage the palms of the hands and the soles of the feet, with extra pressure applied to the tender points. While face-down, medium pressure was applied to the upper shoulder and neck area, and brisk rubbing movements were performed along the spine.

**Assessments** Subjects were informed that assessments were being made on massage effects on the elder volunteers, including self-reports (of anxiety, mood, depression, self-esteem, and daily activities), behavior observations, and stress hormones from urine and saliva samples. On the first (Day 1) and last (Day 21) days of the treatment periods (both the giving massage and receiving massage periods) assessment measures were collected according to the following schedule.

1. Forty-five minutes prior to the massage, saliva and urine were collected from the elder volunteers.

2. Forty minutes prior to the massage, the self-report measures – the Feeling Good Thermometer, Multiple Affect Adjective Check-List, the Center for Epidemiologic Studies–Depression Scale, Duke–UNC Health Profile, and a lifestyle diary – were administered to the elder volunteers.

3. Immediately after the massage the volunteers received two of the self-report measures again (Feeling Good Thermometer and the Multiple Affect Adjective Check-List.

4. Thirty minutes following the massage, saliva samples were taken from the volunteers.

### Pre/post-massage measures (short-term measures)

*The Feeling Good Thermometer.* This is a visual analogue scale for measuring affect (Appendix 1A). The scale ranges from 0 to 10, with a higher temperature reflecting more positive feelings.

*The Multiple Affect Adjective Check-List (MAACL).* This provides a measure of anxiety and depressed mood (Zuckerman & Lubin 1965). The total score is the number of positive items checked plus the number of zero items not checked. Subjects were given the Today form (as opposed to the General form) of the test.

*Saliva samples.* These were collected to assay stress hormone (cortisol) levels. These were obtained by placing a cotton dental swab dipped in sugar-free lemonade crystals along the subject's gumline for 30 seconds. The swab is then placed in a syringe and the saliva is removed and inserted into a microcentrifuge tube for freezing.

### First-day/last-day measures (longer-term measures)

*The Center for Epidemiologic Studies–Depression Scale (CES–D).* This was used to measure depressive symptoms of the elder volunteers (Radloff 1977). The 20-item scale contains items relating to depressed mood and psychophysiologic indicators of depression. Respondents rated how frequently each symptom was experienced during the past week on a 4-point scale. The ratings form a summed score ranging from 0 to 60. A score of 15 is the cutpoint typically used in research samples to indicate depressive symptoms. This cutpoint corresponds to the 80th percentile of scores in community samples. Both the reliability and validity of the CES–D have been supported across demographically diverse subsamples of the general population (Radloff 1977).

*The Duke–UNC Health Profile (DUHP).* This was used to assess four dimensions of health: symptom status and physical, emotional, and social functioning. This 63-item questionnaire has been used to measure adult health status in primary care settings and in health and lifestyle research. Previous research supported the reliability and validity of the DUHP (Parkerson, Gehlbach & Wagner, 1981).

*The Lifestyle Diary.* This was designed specifically for this study to assess changes in

1. *physical activity and health* (number of hours of sleep, naps taken, headaches, medications/prescriptions taken, trips to the doctor's office)
2. *entertainment/leisure* (number of hours of TV watching, phone calls made/received, visitors, sexual activities)
3. *eating and drinking* (number of cups of coffee, alcoholic drinks, cigarettes smoked, meals eaten in/out).

This checklist (Appendix 1B) was completed by the volunteers about their previous weekend activities at the beginning and end of the study. For the purpose of this study, three relevant stress variables were analyzed, including the change across the course of the study in the number of cups of coffee, the number of social phone calls, and the number of doctor's office visits.

*Urine samples.* These were collected from the elder volunteers 45 minutes prior to massage. Urine samples were assayed for longer-term changes in stress hormones (cortisol, norepinephrine, epinephrine, and dopamine).

## Results

Repeated-measures analyses were performed on the self-report data and the biochemical data, with pre/post massage, first-day/last-day, and giving versus receiving as the repeated measures.

**Giving massage** As can be seen in Table 1.13, the analyses suggested the following for giving massage.

For the pre/post massage comparisons:

1. affect improved from pre to post massage on the first and the last day

2. anxiety decreased from pre to post massage on the first and last day
3. depressed mood decreased on the first and last days
4. cortisol levels decreased on the first and last days.

For the first-day/last-day comparisons:

1. depression decreased from the first to the last day
2. the Health Profile scores improved from the first to the last day
3. Lifestyle Diary scores improved: specifically, the number of visits to the doctor and number of cups of coffee decreased and the number of social phone calls increased
4. stress hormone (norepinephrine and epinephrine) levels decreased.

**Receiving massage** For the pre/post receiving massage comparisons:

1. affect improved from pre to post massage but only on the last day
2. depressed mood decreased from pre to post massage but only on the last day. For the first-day/last-day comparisons, depression decreased from the first to last day (see Table 1.14).

**Table 1.13** Means for giving massage therapy (Study 5)

| Variables | First day | | Last day | |
|---|---|---|---|---|
| Pre/post-therapy | Pre | Post | Pre | Post |
| Affect | 7.7 | 8.7* | 8.3 | 9.4* |
| Anxiety | 0.6 | 0.1* | 0.3 | 0.1* |
| Depressed mood | 1.4 | 0.7* | 1.7 | 1.1* |
| Saliva cortisol | 1.9 | 1.3**** | 1.7 | 1.3**** |

| First-day/last-day | First day | Last day |
|---|---|---|
| Depression (CES–D) | 18.2 | 14.3* |
| Health profile | 60.9 | 67.2* |
| Lifestyle diary | 35.9 | 30.9* |
| Norepinephrine | 52.3 | 32.9*** |
| Epinephrine | 14.1 | 7.7**** |
| Dopamine | 330.2 | 279.6 |
| Cortisol | 103.6 | 104.3 |

Pre/post massage session significance levels for the first and last days are indicated by asterisks after the 2nd and after the 4th column means in the top half of the table. Asterisks in the bottom half of the table indicate first-day/last-day significance levels (* $p < 0.05$; ** $p < 0.01$; *** $p < 0.005$; **** $p < 0.001$).

**Table 1.14**   Means for receiving massage therapy (Study 5)

| Variables | First day | | Last day | |
|---|---|---|---|---|
| Pre/post-therapy | Pre | Post | Pre | Post |
| Affect | 8.9 | 9.0 | 8.0 | 8.9* |
| Anxiety | 0.4 | 0.2 | 0.6 | 0.7 |
| Depressed mood | 0.9 | 0.8 | 0.8 | 0.4** |
| Saliva cortisol | 1.5 | 1.2 | 1.1 | 0.8* |
| **First-day/last-day** | **First day** | | **Last day** | |
| Depression (CES–D) | 14.4 | | 11.9** | |
| Health profile | 70.9 | | 74.6 | |
| Lifestyle diary | 36.1 | | 34.4 | |
| Norepinephrine | 48.9 | | 40.7 | |
| Epinephrine | 15.6 | | 13.8 | |
| Dopamine | 310.9 | | 307.2 | |
| Cortisol | 111.5 | | 109.9 | |

Pre/post massage sessions significance levels for the first and last days are indicated by asterisks after the and after the 4th column means in the top half of the table. Asterisks in the bottom half of the table indicate first-day/last-day significance levels (* $p < 0.05$, ** $p < 0.01$).

## Discussion

Although several studies have documented the positive effects of massage therapy on depression and stress hormones (Field et al 1992, Ironson et al 1996), this study was the first to measure the benefits for the 'massage therapist'. As expected, this study showed that elder volunteers benefitted from giving massage therapy. The elder volunteers were immediately affected by massaging the infants, as evidenced by their improved affect, their decreased anxiety and depressed mood, and their decreased stress hormone (salivary cortisol) levels. The decreased stress levels probably contributed to their decreased depression over the 3-week period, their lifestyle changes (including drinking less coffee, and increased social calls), and their improved health (making fewer trips to the doctor's office). The decreased stress hormones (cortisol and catecholamine levels) would predictably lead to enhanced immune function (Ironson et al 1996).

These positive effects may relate to contact comfort, as in pet therapy, and enhanced wellbeing, by having a structured activity involving social responsibility. Presumably both of these mechanisms were operating, inasmuch as fewer positive effects were noted over the 3-week period when the same volunteers were receiving massage therapy. For that treatment period the positive effects were only noted on the last day of the study. The fewer effects noted for receiving massage may have related to the elder volunteers feeling 'awkward about the initial massage sessions', nothing that they had 'never been touched in that way.' Thus, the initial anxiety about being massaged may have attenuated the expected immediate effects of receiving massage therapy.

Future studies might explore the combined effects of giving and receiving massage therapy. In addition, assaying immune function would be an important additional measure insofar as waning immune function is a problem at this age. Further, cost–benefit analysis would help demonstrate the cost-effectiveness of massage therapy benefitting both groups of people (the elder retired volunteers and the infants) at the same time. If the value of massage therapy for the giver, and specifically for elder volunteers, is confirmed in future studies with larger samples and with control groups (missing from this exploratory study), then this service might be adopted for elders and for infants to enhance their health and wellbeing.

REFERENCES

Acolet D, Modi N, Giannakoulopoulos X, Bond C, Weg W, Clow A, Glover V 1993 Changes in plasma cortisol and catecholamine concentrations in response to massage in preterm infants. Archives of Diseases of the Child 68:29–31

Armstrong FD, Seidel JF, Swales TP 1983 Pediatric HIV infection: a neuropsychological and educational challenge. Journal of Learning Disabilities 26:92–103

Auckett AD 1981 Baby massage. Newmarket Press, New York

Barnard KE, Bee HL 1983 The impact of temporally patterned stimulation on the development of preterm infants. Child Development 54:1156–1167

Barnes DM 1986 Brain function decline in children with AIDS. Science 232:1196

Beck AT, Ward CH, Mendelson M, Mach JE, Erbaugh J 1961 An inventory for measuring depression. Archives of General Psychiatry 4:561–571

Belman AL 1990 AIDS and pediatric neurology. Neurological Clinics 8:571–603

Belman AL, Diamond G, Dickson D et al 1988 Pediatric acquired immunodeficiency syndrome. American Journal of Diseases in Children 142:29–35

Blanche S, Rouzioux C, Moscato ML et al 1989 A prospective study of infants born to women seropositive for human immunodeficiency virus Type 1. New England Journal of Medicine 320:1643–1648

Brazelton TB 1973 Neonatal behavioral assessment scale. London, Spastic International Medical Publications

Burkett G, Yasin S, Palow D 1990 Perinatal implications of cocaine exposure. Journal of Reproductive Medicine 35:35–42

Center for Disease Control 1989 Update: Acquired immunodeficiency syndrome–United States. Morbidity and Mortality Weekly 39:81–86

Cohn JF, Matias R, Tronick EZ, Connell D, Lyons-Ruth K 1986 Face-to-face interactions of depressed mothers and their infants. In: Tronick EZ, Field T (eds) Maternal depression and infant disturbance, Jossey-Bass, San Francisco, pp 31–45

Coles CD, Platzman KA, Smith IE et al 1990 Effects of maternal use of cocaine and alcohol on neonatal behavior. Paper presented at the International Conference on Infant Studies, Montreal, April 1990

Costello EJ, Edelbrock CS, Costello AJ 1985 Validity of the NIMH Diagnostic Interview Schedule for Children: a comparison between psychiatric and pediatric referrals. Journal of Abnormal Child Psychology 13:579–595

Curless RG 1989 Congenital AIDS: review of neurological problems. Child's Nervous System 5:9–11

Dixon WJ, Brown MB (eds) 1979 BMDP-79: Biomedical Computer Programs P-Series. University of California Press, Berkeley CA

Dubowitz LMS, Dubowitz V, Goldberg C 1970 Clinical assessment of gestational age in the newborn infant. Journal of Pediatrics 111:571–578

Eisen L, Field T, Bandstra E, Roberts J, Morrow C, Larson S 1991 Perinatal cocaine effects on neonatal stress behavior and performance on the Brazelton scale. Pediatrics 88:477–480

Field T 1980 Supplemental stimulation of preterm neonates. Early Human Development 4:301–314

Field T 1984 Early interactions between infants and their postpartum depressed mothers. Infant Behavior and Development 7:517–522

Field T 1992 Infants of depressed mothers. Development and Psychopathology 4:49–66

Field T, Schanberg S 1990 Massage enhances growth in preterm neonates. In: Brazelton B, Field T (eds) Advances in touch. Johnson & Johnson, Skillman NJ

Field T, Dempsey J, Shuman HH 1984 Five-year follow-up of preterm respiratory distress syndrome and postterm postmaturity syndrome infants. In: Field T, Sostek A (eds) Infants born at risk: physiological, perceptual and cognitive processes. Grune & Stratton, New York, pp 317–335

Field T, Schanberg SM, Scafidi F et al 1986 Tactile/kinesthetic stimulation effects on preterm neonates. Pediatrics 77:654–658

Field T, Scafidi F, Schanberg S 1987 Massage of preterm newborns to improve growth and development. Pediatric Nursing 13:385–387

Field T, Morrow C, Valdeon C, Larson S, Kuhn C, Schanberg S 1992 Massage reduces anxiety in child and adolescent psychiatric patients. Journal of the American Academy of Child and Adolescent Psychiatry 31:125–131

Field T, Grizzle N, Scafidi F, Schanberg S 1996 Massage and relaxation therapies' effects on depressed adolescent mothers. Adolescence 31:903–911

Field T, Ironson G, Pickens J, Nawrocki T, Fox N, Scafidi F, Burman I, Schanberg S 1996 Massage therapy reduces anxiety and enhances EEG pattern of alertness and math computations. International Journal of Neuroscience 86:197–205

Grossberg J, Alf E, Jr 1985 Interaction with pet dogs: effects on human cardiovascular response. Journal of the Delta Society 12:20–27

Hadeed AJ, Siegel SR 1989 Maternal cocaine use during pregnancy: effect on the newborn infant. Pediatrics 84:205–210

Hendrie H, Crosset J 1990 An overview of depression in the elderly. Psychiatric Annals 20:64–69

Ironson G, Field T, Scafidi F et al 1996 Massage therapy is associated with enhancement of the immune system's cytotoxic capacity. International Journal of Neuroscience 84:205–218

Johnson JP, Nair P, Hines SE 1989 Natural history and serological diagnosis of infants born to human immunodeficiency virus-infected women. American Journal of Diseases in Children 143:1147–1153

Kilbourne BW, Buehler JW, Rogers MF 1990 AIDS as a cause of death in children, adolescents, and young adults. American Journal of Public Health 80:499–500

Kletter R, Jeremy RJ, Rumsey C, Weintraub P, Cowan M 1989 A prospective study of mental and motor development of infants born to HIV infected intravenous drug abusing mothers [abstract]. V International Conference on AIDS: Abstracts vol 5:225

Kuhn C, Schanberg S, Field T et al 1991 Tactile/kinesthetic stimulation effects on sympathetic and adrenocortical function in preterm infants. Journal of Pediatrics 119:434–440

Lester BM, Als H, Brazelton TB 1982 Regional obstetric anesthesia and newborn behavior: a reanalysis toward synergistic effects. Child Development 53:687–692

Littman D, Parmelee A 1978 Medical correlates of infant development. Pediatrics 61:470–474

McCullough P 1991 Geriatric depression: a typical presentation, hidden meaning. Geriatrics 46:72–76

Meaney MJ, Aitken DH, Bhatnagar M, Bodnoff SR, Mitchell JB, Sarrieau A 1990 Neonatal handling and the development of the adrenocortical response to stress. In: Brazelton B, Field T (eds) Advances in touch. Johnson & Johnson, Skillman NJ

Mittleman G, Valenstein ES 1984 Ingestive behavior evoked by hypothalamic stimulation and schedule-induced polydipsia are related. Science 27:415–420

Modi N, Glover J 1996 Massage therapy for preterm infants. Paper presented at Touch Research Symposium, Providence, Rhode Island

Mussachia XJ, Deavers DR, Meininger GA et al 1980 A model for hypokinesis: Effects on muscle atrophy in the rat. Journal of Applied Physiology 48:479–485

Myers JL 1979 Fundamentals of experimental design. Allyn & Bacon, Boston

Ottenbacher KJ, Muller L, Brandt D, Heintzelman A, Hojem P, Sharpe P 1987 The effectiveness of tactile stimulation as a form of early intervention: a quantitative evaluation. Journal of Developmental and Behavioral Pediatrics 8:68–76

Parkerson G, Gehlbach S, Wagner E 1981 The Duke–UNC Health Profile. Med Care 19:806–828

Peckham CS, Tedder RS, Briggs M et al 1990 Prevalence of maternal HIV infection based on unlinked anonymous testing of newborn babies. Lancet 19:561–569

Porges SW 1985 Method and apparatus for evaluating rhythmic oscillations in aperiodic response systems. United States Patent no. 4510944

Powell GF, Brasel JA, Blizzard RM 1967 Emotional deprivation and growth retardation simulating idiopathic hypopituitarism. New England Journal of Medicine 276:1271–1276

Radloff L 1977 The CES-D scale: a self-report depression scale for research in the general population. Applied Psychological Measures 1:385–401

Rausch PB 1981 Effects of tactile and kinesthetic stimulation on premature infants. Journal of Obstetric Gynecologic Neonatal Nursing 10:34

Richards IS, Kulkarni AP, Bremner WF 1990 Cocaine-induced arrhythmia in human fetal myocardium in vitro: possible mechanism for fetal death. Pharmacological Toxicology 66:150–154

Rosenak D, Diamont Z, Yaffe H et al 1990 Maternal use during pregnancy and its effect on the mother, fetus, and the infant. Obstetrics & Gynecology Survey 45:348–359

Rowe DC, Plomin R 1977 Temperament in early childhood. Journal of Personality Assessment 41:150–156

Ruegg R, Zisook S, Swerdlow M 1988 Depression in the aged: an overview. Psychiatric Clinics of North America 11:83–108

Scafidi F, Field T 1996 Massage therapy improves behavior in neonates born to HIV positive mothers. Journal of Pediatric Psychology 21:889–898

Scafidi F, Field T, Schanberg S, Bauer C, Vega-Lahr N, Garcia R 1986 Effects of tactile/kinesthetic stimulation on the clinical course and sleep/wake behavior of preterm neonates. Infant Behavior and Development 9:91–105

Scafidi FA, Field TM, Schanberg SM et al 1990 Massage stimulates growth in preterm infants: a replication. Infant Behavior and Development 13:167–188

Scafidi F, Field T, Wheeden A et al 1996 Behavioral and hormonal differences in preterm neonates exposed to cocaine in vitro. Pediatrics 97:851–855

Schaeffer M, Hatcher RP, Barglow PD 1980 Prematurity and infant stimulation: a review of research. Child Psychiatry Human Development 10:199–212

Schanberg S 1995 Genetic basis for touch effects. In: Field T (ed) Touch in early development. Lawrence Erlbaum, Hillsdale NJ

Schanberg S, Field T 1987 Sensory deprivation stress and supplemental stimulation in the rat pup and preterm human neonate. Child Development 58:1431–1447

Schanberg SM, Evoniuk G, Kuhn CM 1984 Tactile and nutritional aspects of maternal care: specific regulators of neuroendocrine function and cellular development. Processes of Social Experimental Biological Medicine 175:135–139

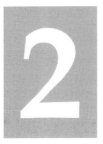

# Pain reduction during painful procedures and chronic pain syndromes

Different types of tactile, auditory and olfactory stimulation such as massage, music and aroma therapies appear to reduce pain or to reduce perception of pain. Although the underlying mechanisms are unclear, there are many empirical examples of massage therapy effects, including the reduction of pain during painful procedures such as labor for childbirth and skin brushing for removing debris from burns and for the reduction of pain in syndromes such as juvenile rheumatoid arthritis, fibromyalgia, lower back pain and migraine headaches.

## PAINFUL PROCEDURES

### Study 1: Labor in childbirth

In many countries pregnant women are massaged several times daily for relaxation and to reduce their anxiety levels. Touch and massage have been used during labor in nearly every culture for hundreds of years (Hedstrom & Newton 1986). Only recently has physical support been available to Western women during delivery (Kennell et al 1991). In the past, massage and support during labor were used to improve or correct the position of the fetus, to stimulate uterine contractions, to prevent the fetus from rising back up in the abdomen, and to exert mechanical pressure to aid in the expulsion of the child (Engelman 1982). However, today the focus tends to center more on relaxation to reduce anxiety and alleviate pain (Hedstrom & Newton 1986).

A strong association between maternal anxiety (typically measured by self-report questionnaires) and labor discomfort has been reported. Labor discomfort is thought to arise from fear of the unknown, which leads to sympathetic arousal producing tension in the circular fibers of the uterus and rigidity at the opening of the cervix (Read 1972). This force acts against the expulsive muscle fibers in labor, producing tension within the uterine cavity, which is interpreted by the laboring mother as pain. Prolonged uterine muscle tension can produce ischemia (local and temporary anemia due to poor blood flow), resulting in pain. Maternal anxiety can cause increased levels of catecholamines, resulting in a decrease in uterine contractility and blood flow, and therefore in pain and maternal complications during delivery (Kennell et al 1991).

Prenatal classes often include instructions on visualization and imagery, with the expectation that women will be more relaxed and in control of pain during labor. A recent study on the effectiveness of imagery, however, failed to find differences between women who participated in visual imagery training sessions and a control group with regard to self-reports on anxiety and pain levels during labor (Korol & Von Baeyer 1992). However, when intense visual imagery training sessions were used in the management of labor pain and other chronic pain conditions (Brown 1984, Lindberg & Lawlis 1988, Raft, Smith & Warren 1986) the results were more favorable. Thus, visual imagery techniques may be effective for reducing pain associated with labor, but at the cost of extensive training.

Being touched in general during labor and delivery is perceived by mothers as a positive experience (Stolte 1976). For example, abdominal massage used in some Lamaze childbirth educational classes has been suggested for easing discomfort of tired or cramping muscles and facilitating control and relaxation during labor (Wideman & Singer 1984). The presence and involvement of partners who touch the women during labor have been significantly correlated with less need for drugs, shorter labors, fewer perinatal problems and more optimal maternal interactions (Sosa et al 1980).

Studies involving doulas (labor support people) who have already experienced a labor of their own and remain at the patient's bedside from time of admission to the end of birth show a positive impact on labor (Kennell et al 1991). Studies involving male partners, such as the husband, have also reported positive effects (Bertsch et al 1990). In a study comparing doulas and male partners, doulas touched the laboring women more and were present for more time during labor than male partners (Bertsch et al 1990). A pilot study by Kennell and his colleagues (Nagashima et al 1987) reported inconclusive results when examining male partner behavior during labor and delivery, with some partners providing excellent support while others did not.

These reports combined suggest that persons providing more touch have been more favorably viewed by women in labor. The touching seems to reduce maternal anxiety and facilitate labor and delivery. However, it is still unclear whether the reduced anxiety and pain derive from the supportive presence of another person, such as the doula, or whether active touch such as massage therapy could further reduce those problems. The present study compared partners massaging women in labor versus the partners being present and simply doing what came naturally during labor (typically the coaching in breathing exercises they had learned in prenatal classes). We expected that massage coupled with the breathing exercises would have more positive effects than the breathing exercises alone on anxiety and pain as well as length of labor.

## Method

**Sample**  The sample was comprised of 28 middle SES women (mean age = 29.7) who were recruited from Lamaze classes during their last trimester (mean = 37 weeks gestation). The women were most frequently married (91%) and were distributed 34% White, 9% Black, and 57% Hispanic. Other sample characteristics were: (1) 74% had worked through the 7th month of pregnancy; (2) 75% had more than 12 prenatal visits; (3) 60% had attended 1–6 childbirth classes, 63% had learned the breathing techniques and 60% reported using the breathing techniques during delivery; (4) 67% reported having had a massage previously. The women were randomly assigned (based on a table of numbers) to a massage therapy or a control group. The groups did not differ on any of the above baseline variables. The groups also did not differ on the relationship with labor partner (88% were husbands, 9% parents, and 3% relatives).

**Procedures**

*Massage therapy group.* Following the admissions interview the massage was taught to the partner for a mean of 10 minutes by a massage therapist. At approximately 3–5 cm cervical dilation, the subjects then received 20 minutes of head, shoulder/back, hand, and foot massage. The massage entailed moderate pressure and smooth movements specifically adapted to relax the strained and

stressed areas of the laboring body. The 20-minute sequence consisted of smooth, timed, clockwise circular stroking movements
for 5-minute consecutive periods in each of the four regions while
the mother was lying on her side: (1) around the head, down the
temple to the (2) neck and shoulder, across and down the back (3)
to the hand and (4) then down to the foot. The same 20-minute
massage was repeated by the partner every hour for 5 hours. The
massage therapist was present only until the partner felt comfortable giving the massage on his/her own. None of the partners
refused to give the massage and none of them reported being
uncomfortable delivering the massage. Immediately after the first
massage the research associate who was blind to group assignment was allowed into the labor room to record measures on the
immediate effects of the massage.

*Attention control group.* The control subjects and their partners
were simply asked to engage in whatever activities they had
been taught – for example, the breathing coaching – or whatever
came naturally during labor. Their activities were observed by
a research associate who served not only as a control for the
subject receiving extra attention but also to record whether anyone
in the control group was receiving massage. None of the control
group mothers requested or received massage from their partners,
even though 60% had been previously exposed to massage. The
same baseline and follow-up assessments were conducted at the
same time as those of the massage group (a pre/post 20-minute
interval).

*Self-report measures.* Childbirth labor was considered to be
that time period from the onset of hospitalization until the patient
was taken to the delivery room at full cervical dilation. As
soon as the subject was admitted to the hospital, a demographic
interview was conducted to ensure comparability of the two
groups.

*Demographic information* included maternal age, ethnicity, marital
status, socioeconomic status, prenatal care, attendance at childbirth
classes, self-report measures on importance of touch and previous
experience being massaged.

*Pre/post-massage measures*

• *The Profile of Mood States Depression Scale* (POMS) (McNair,
Lorr & Droppleman 1971), a 14-item Likert-type self-report questionnaire of adjectives describing current depressed mood, was
completed by the mothers before and after the massage session.
• *Feeling Good Thermometer* (Appendix 1A) was used to assess
in a less cognitive way the mother's feeling of wellbeing.

• *Stress Level and Labor Pains.* The mothers rated their stress levels and labor pains before and after the massage on a 5-point Likert scale.

• *Partners' Report Measures.* Each partner rated the mother's stress level and labor progression on 5-point Likert scales before and after the massage.

• *The Behavior Observation Scale* (BOS) (Platania-Solazzo et al 1992). Before and after the massage session the mother's behavior was rated by an observer blind to the mother's group status on a 3-point continuum on four scales, including activity, anxiety, and positive facial expressions.

### Post-labor measures

• *The Center for Epidemiological Studies Scale for Depression* (CES–D) (Radloff 1977) was used to assess depressed mood.

• *The Touch Sensitivity Scale* (Royeen 1987) was used to document the mothers' sensitivity to tactile stimulation. This scale includes 22 items on reactions to different types of touch, including whether the individual finds being accidentally touched aversive.

• *Labor and neonatal measures.* The hospital records were then examined by a research assistant who was blind to the mother's group assignment. The following data were recorded: hours of labor, days of hospitalization, the infant's gestational age, birth weight, length, head circumference, Ponderal Index, and perinatal data on the Obstetric and Postnatal Complications Scales (Littman & Parmelee 1978).

## Results

Data analyses on the self-report measures revealed the following (see Table 2.1).

1. The massage group mothers versus the control group mothers reported less depressed mood (on the POMS), feeling better (on the visual analogue thermometer), lower stress levels, and decreased labor pains.

2. the control group mothers reported increased labor pains across the same period of time. The massage versus control group partners reported lower maternal stress levels and greater labor progression.

Data analyses on the behavior observation measures suggested the following (see Table 2.2).

**Table 2.1** Means for self-report and partner's measures for pre/post-labor massage/control sessions (Study 1)

|  | Pre | | Post | |
|---|---|---|---|---|
|  | Massage | Control | Massage | Control |
| *Self-report measures* |  |  |  |  |
| Depressed mood (POMS) | 14.0 | 14.4 | 6.9* | 14.9 |
| Feeling Good Thermometer[1] | 5.6 | 6.5 | 6.8* | 6.6 |
| Stress level | 3.3 | 3.4 | 5.2** | 3.5 |
| Labor pains | 5.0 | 4.3 | 3.5* | 5.0* |
| *Partners' report measures* |  |  |  |  |
| Mothers' stress level[1] | 3.4 | 3.3 | 5.4* | 3.6 |
| Labor progression[1] | 3.7 | 4.1 | 4.1* | 3.7* |

[1] High values are optimal.
Asterisks denote group differences (* $p < 0.05$; ** $p < 0.001$).

**Table 2.2** Means for observer measures for pre/post-labor massage/control sessions (Study 1)

| Behavior observation measures | Pre | | Post | |
|---|---|---|---|---|
|  | Massage | Control | Massage | Control |
| Activity[1] | 1.7 | 1.9 | 2.5*** | 2.0 |
| Anxiety[1] | 1.9 | 1.8 | 2.4** | 1.8 |
| Positive facial expressions[1] | 1.9 | 2.0 | 2.3* | 2.6* |

[1] High values are optimal.
Asterisks denote group differences (* $p < 0.05$; ** $p < 0.01$; *** $p < 0.001$).

1. The massage group showed lower activity and anxiety levels and more positive facial expressions after the massage.

2. the control group showed more positive facial expressions following a similar time period.

Data analyses on the post-labor variables suggested the following effects favoring the massage group (see Table 2.3).

1. less touch sensitivity
2. lower levels of perinatal depression
3. fewer hours in labor
4. a shorter hospital stay.

*Discussion*

Data from three different sources (the mother, partner and observer) converged to suggest that massage therapy reduced stress and pain during labor. The pregnant women themselves reported less depressed mood state, feeling better, having less stress and fewer labor pains following massage. In contrast, labor pains increased

**Table 2.3** Means for post-labor measures

| Post-labor measures | Massage | Control |
|---|---|---|
| Postpartum depression (CES–D) | 15.4 | 19.8* |
| Touch sensitivity | 27.9 | 11.1* |
| # hours in labor | 8.5 | 11.3* |
| # days hospital stay | 1.3 | 2.2* |

Asterisk denotes group differences (* $p < 0.05$).

in those women who were not massaged. The mothers' partners (most frequently their husbands) also evaluated the massaged women as being less stressed, and their labor progressed better, following the massage sessions. Behavioral observations by an observer who was blind to the women's group assignment rated the women as having lower activity and anxiety levels. The only similarity between the groups was an increase in positive facial expressions.

Lower levels of self-reported stress and depressed mood state and decreased behavioral anxiety have been reported following massage therapy in several studies (Field et al 1992, Field, Ironson et al 1996). These lower anxiety/stress levels have typically been associated with lower stress hormone (cortisol) levels. Lower pain levels have also resulted from massage therapy given to adults with pain syndromes such as fibromyalgia (Sunshine et al 1996). The underlying mechanism for reduced stress hormones is unclear, although we have speculated elsewhere that reduced anxiety and stress hormones may be mediated by increasing parasympathetic activity accompanying massage. The mechanism underlying reduced pain is also unclear. Some investigators speculate that pressure stimulation from massage pre-empts the processing of pain stimulation because pressure fibers are longer and more myelinated and thus can relay the signal to the brain faster than pain fibers (Melzack & Wall 1965). That these immediate effects of massage therapy translated into longer-term effects, including shorter labor, shorter hospital stay, less touch sensitivity and less postpartum depression, was more surprising.

These findings are tempered by the fact that the women's self-reports might have been influenced by their wish to please their partners following the massage and by the partners who provided the massage also providing their assessment on at least two measures. In addition, the sample was small, suggesting the need for studies on larger samples and more comprehensive labor outcome measures. Having a larger sample size might reveal effects on neonatal outcome. Nonetheless, these data highlight the cost-effectiveness of significant others providing massage during labor. Further research is needed on the underlying mechanisms and whether neonatal outcome can be enhanced by providing massage therapy during pregnancy long before the onset of labor.

## Study 2: Massage therapy prior to debridement for burn patients

Massage therapy has also been used to reduce anticipatory anxiety prior to debridement (skin brushing to remove debris from severe burns) and to indirectly alleviate pain during that procedure (Field, Peck et al 1998). After a 5-day course of 30-minute massages prior to debridement, burn patients had lower depression and anxiety levels and associated decreases in stress hormones (cortisol), probably because of the decrease in pain.

Many burn patients feel that the treatment for burn is more painful than the burn itself (Andreasen, Noyes & Hartford 1972). Procedural pain during wound cleaning and debridement is described as short in duration but intense. Burn patients also experience depression and anxiety which in turn affect the patient's perception of pain (Patterson 1992). If these feelings can be reduced or controlled, the patient's perception of pain can also be reduced.

Various therapies such as transcutaneous electrical nerve stimulation (TENS) (Kimball et al 1987), electromyographic biofeedback (EMG) (Achterberg, Kenner & Lawlis 1988), and hypnosis have been tried for pain, with varying degrees of success (Gilboa et al 1990). Studies have demonstrated that TENS can reduce pain in burn patients (Kimball et al 1987), EMG biofeedback assists muscle relaxation and manipulation, and a combination of relaxation therapy, mental imagery, and EMG biofeedback has been noted to reduce pain and anxiety (Achterberg et al 1988). Massage therapy has not yet been tried with burn patients, although it might be expected to have positive effects on pain and anxiety/ depression levels. For example, massage has been associated with reduced pain in fibromyalgia patients (Sunshine et al 1996) and with reduced depression and anxiety as well as improved sleep patterns in depressed psychiatric patients (Field et al 1992). In the latter study, massage therapy also reduced stress hormones, specifically cortisol and norepinephrine. Consistent with these findings, massage therapy was expected to reduce pain, anxiety, depressed mood state and stress hormones in burn patients prior to debridement and to reduce their resting pain, anxiety, and depression across the 1-week treatment period.

*Method*

**Sample** Twenty-eight adult burn patients were recruited consecutively as they were admitted to our Burn Center. The subjects were distributed 86% male, and they were 41% Hispanic, 30% Black, and 29% Non-Hispanic White. Thirty-six percent were married, 29% had some college education, 69% were employed, 38% had an income greater than $20 000, 58% were visited often by family and friends, and 71% had never had a massage. On average the burn size was 10%, and the patients were recruited for the study on average 9 days after they had been burned. The subjects were randomly assigned to a massage therapy or a standard treatment control group. The two groups did not differ on the above background variables.

Routine care of burn patients at our Burn Center was given to all subjects. After admission, wound care and debridement were done twice daily using a combination of narcotic analgesics and benzodiazepine sedatives for comfort. Silver sulfadiazine cream was applied to the wounds to reduce bacterial colonization. Deep second and third degree burns were excised and grafted within 10 days of injury.

**Procedure**

*Standard treatment.* During the study period all burn patients continued to receive their standard medical care, which included physician examinations, medications and physical therapy. Narcotics and benzodiazepines were routinely used to improve comfort levels.

*Massage therapy.* The massage therapy group subjects, in addition, received a 20-minute massage once a day for 1 week. The massage sessions were held just prior to the early morning (9 a.m.) debridement sessions. The massage session was comprised of two standard phases. The first phase began with the subject in a supine position. The massage therapist stroked five regions of the body (face, chest, stomach, legs, and arms) using moderate pressure stroking (Fig. 2.1). For the second phase, the subject was in a prone position and the subject's back was massaged.

*Assessments.* Subjects were assessed on the effects of massage therapy before and after their early morning (9 a.m.) massage sessions (or before and after 20 minutes of sitting and relaxing in the control group) on the first and last days of the study period. The pre/post-therapy measures included the *State Trait Anxiety Inventory (STAI)* (Spielberger, Gorsuch & Lushene 1970), behavior observations of the subjects and the subjects' pulse, and the saliva samples provided by the subjects for cortisol assays. The same measures were collected after the sessions on the first and last days of the study. Longer-term effects were assessed by three pain

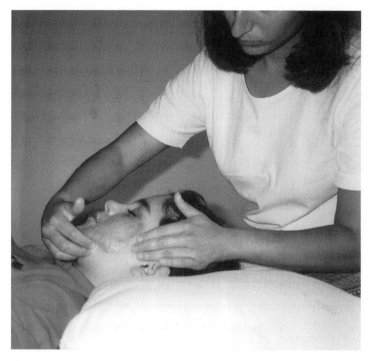

**Figure 2.1** Burn patient receiving massage.

measures (The McGill Pain Questionnaire, the Present Pain Intensity, and the Visual Analogue Scale) and the Profile of Moods State (depression, anger, and vigor) on the first and last days of the study (Spielberger et al 1970).

*Assessments of immediate effects (pre/post-session measures)*

• *State Trait Anxiety Inventory (STAI)* measures how the subject feels right now on 40 items with answer choices of 1 = not at all / almost never, 2 = somewhat/sometimes, 3 = moderately so / often, and 4 = very much so / almost always.

• The *Behavior Observation Scale* (Platania-Solazzo et al 1992) was completed.

• *Radial pulse rates* were taken for 30 seconds prior to and after the massage session.

• *Salivary cortisol samples* were collected prior to and 20 minutes after the massage at the same time of day each day (9 a.m.). Due to the 20-minute lag in cortisol change, saliva samples were collected 20 minutes following the session. Saliva was obtained by placing sugar-free lemonade crystals on a cotton dental swab and placing the swab in the subject's mouth for 30 seconds. The swab was then placed in a syringe, and a plunger was depressed to insert the saliva into a tube. Samples were assayed for cortisol levels by Dr Saul Schanberg at Duke University Medical School.

### Assessments of longer-term effects (first-day/last-day measures)

• The *McGill Pain Questionnaire* (Melzack 1987) defines the sensory, affective, and evaluative dimensions of pain based on a four point Likert scale. The questionnaire consists of eleven questions based on the sensory dimensions of pain and four questions based on the affective dimensions of pain, with answer choices of 0 = none, 1 = mild, 2 = moderate, and 3 = severe.

• The evaluative dimension of pain is determined by a *Present Pain Intensity (PPI)* and a *Visual Analogue Scale (VAS)*. The PPI scale measures pain experienced right now based on a 6-point Likert scale with choices of 0 = no pain, 1 = mild, 2 = discomforting, 3 = distressing, 4 = horrible, and 5 = excruciating. The VAS is a no pain to worst possible pain rating.

• The *Profile of Mood States* (McNair et al 1971) was also completed.

## Results

**Immediate effects (pre/post-session measures)** Data analyses suggested that the massage therapy group, compared with the control group, immediately benefitted from the massage in several ways (see Tables 2.4 and 2.5):

1. On both days 1 and 5 of the treatment period, their state anxiety scores were lower following the massage therapy session.

2. On both the first and last days, their behavior observation ratings improved after massage for all behaviors (except co-operation), including affect, activity, vocalizations, and anxiety.

3. On both days, their saliva cortisol levels decreased following the massage.

4. On both the first and last days, both the massage and resting groups' pulses decreased after their sessions.

**Longer-term effects (first-day/last-day measures)** Data analyses of the longer-term effects suggested that the massage therapy group benefitted more than the control group over the longer term as follows.

1. Pain ratings were lower, including McGill Pain, Present Pain Intensity and Visual Analogue Scale ratings.

**Table 2.4**  Immediate and longer-term measures of massage therapy effects on burn patients (Study 2)

|  | First day | | Last day | |
|---|---|---|---|---|
|  | Pre | Post | Pre | Post |
| *Immediate (pre/post) measures* | | | | |
| *State Anxiety* | 44.9$_a$ | 32.4$_b$**** | 43.2$_a$ | 34.9$_b$**** |
| *Behavior ratings* | | | | |
| Affect | 2.7$_a$ | 1.8$_b$**** | 2.3$_c$ | 1.6$_b$*** |
| Activity[1] | 1.9$_a$ | 2.9$_b$**** | 2.3$_c$ | 2.8$_b$* |
| Vocalization | 2.2$_a$ | 1.3$_b$**** | 2.1$_a$ | 1.5$_b$**** |
| Anxiety[1] | 1.9$_a$ | 2.8$_b$**** | 2.3$_c$ | 2.9$_b$**** |
| Cooperation | 2.7$_a$ | 2.6$_a$ | 2.7$_a$ | 2.6$_a$ |
| *Pulse* | 93.8$_a$ | 88.0$_b$**** | 80.1$_c$ | 75.6$_d$*** |
| *Saliva cortisol* | 3.5$_a$ | 2.4$_b$*** | 2.8$_c$ | 2.3$_b$* |
| *Longer-term (first-day/last-day) measures* | | | | |
| McGill Pain | 23.6$_a$ | | 16.0$_b$** | |
| Present Pain Intensity | 3.2$_a$ | | 1.7$_b$**** | |
| Visual Analogue Scale | 5.3$_a$ | | 3.8$_b$** | |
| *Profile of Mood States* | | | | |
| Depression | 16.1$_a$ | | 10.7$_b$** | |
| Anger | 11.1$_a$ | | 5.6$_b$* | |
| Vigor | 10.3$_a$ | | 10.9$_a$ | |

[1] Higher score is optimal.
Asterisks denote significant differences at: * $p < 0.05$; ** $p < 0.01$; *** $p < 0.005$; **** $p < 0.001$.
Different subscript letters denote significant differences.

    2. Profile of Mood state ratings were more improved, including depression and anger ratings.

    3. Behavior ratings improved more over the 5-day period, including state, activity, and anxiety.

    4. Resting pulse was lower on the last day of treatment.

    5. Salivary cortisol was lower on the last day of treatment.

## Discussion

The decreases in state anxiety and cortisol levels immediately after the massage therapy sessions were not surprising, inasmuch as decreased anxiety and cortisol levels have occurred in virtually all massage therapy studies (Field et al 1992, Ironson et al 1996). Having the behavior ratings going in the same direction, with state, activity, vocalization, and anxiety ratings improving and pulse decreasing after massage, provides confirmatory behavioral data for the self-report state anxiety scores and for the salivary cortisol levels.

**Table 2.5**    Immediate and longer-term measures for control group (Study 2)

|  | First day | | Last day | |
|---|---|---|---|---|
|  | Pre | Post | Pre | Post |
| *Immediate (pre/post) measures* | | | | |
| *State Anxiety* | 39.3$_a$ | 39.0$_a$ | 39.8$_a$ | 39.4$_a$ |
| *Behavior ratings* | | | | |
| State | 2.4$_a$ | 2.2$_a$ | 2.3$_a$ | 2.4$_a$ |
| Activity[1] | 1.9$_a$ | 2.5$_b$ | 2.1$_a$ | 2.0$_a$ |
| Vocalization | 2.3$_a$ | 2.0$_a$ | 2.4$_a$ | 2.3$_s$ |
| Anxiety[1] | 1.8$_a$ | 2.0$_a$ | 2.0$_a$ | 1.9$_a$ |
| Cooperation | 2.5$_a$ | 2.6$_a$ | 2.7$_a$ | 2.7$_a$ |
| Pulse | 89.5$_a$ | 87.1$_b$* | 91.6$_a$ | 84.8$_b$* |
| Saliva cortisol | 3.4$_a$ | 3.1$_a$ | 2.9$_a$ | 2.8$_a$ |
| *Longer-term (first-day/last-day)* *measures* | | | | |
| McGill Pain | 23.5$_a$ | | 23.2$_a$ | |
| Present Pain Intensity | 3.6$_a$ | | 3.2$_a$ | |
| Visual Analogue Scale | 4.8$_a$ | | 4.5$_a$ | |
| *Profile of Mood States* | | | | |
| Depression | 17.5$_a$ | | 17.4$_a$ | |
| Anger | 13.2$_a$ | | 13.7$_a$ | |
| Vigor | 12.5$_a$ | | 12.1$_a$ | |

[1] Higher score is optimal.
Asterisks denote significant differences at: * $p < 0.05$; ** $p < 0.01$; *** $p < 0.005$; **** $p < 0.001$.
Different subscript letters denote significant differences.

The significant decrease in pain over the treatment period on as many as three different measures is perhaps more surprising given that the burn conditions were still severe and the painful debridement procedures were still being conducted. The accompanying decrease in depression and anger on the POMS, and the improvement in state, activity, and anxiety behavior ratings, may have contributed to the reduction in pain or vice versa.

Massage therapy involves stimulation of tactile and pressure receptors, which are noted to be longer and more myelinated (insulated) than pain fibers. The gate theory, i.e. longer fibers conveying stimulation to the brain faster and thus 'gating' pain signals, may be operating here (Wall & Melzack 1984). A similar interpretation has been made for TENS, which is thought to provide counter-irritation that interferes with pain pathways (Kimball et al 1987). Others have suggested that simply reducing anxiety and depression can alter the patient's pain perception, potentially elevating the person's threshold (Patterson 1992). Higher thresholds would enable more effective debridement sessions and in turn contribute to faster clinical improvement.

Whatever mechanisms are involved, the short-term reduction in stress/anxiety would facilitate debridement sessions, and the long-term decrease in depression would certainly contribute to a better clinical course. As in our study on pain reduction in fibromyalgia patients (Sunshine et al 1996), the pain reduction and decreased depression were strongly related. Further research is needed on the underlying mechanisms explaining the relationship between massage therapy and pain reduction and on the various parameters of massage therapy to determine their relative effectiveness (e.g. tactile and pressure stimulation) and how long the benefits persist and whether a steady dose of massage therapy is needed for pain alleviation in burn patients.

## PAIN SYNDROMES

Noting significant pain reduction following painful procedures suggested that massage therapy might also alleviate pain in chronic conditions such as juvenile rheumatoid arthritis, fibromyalgia, premenstrual syndrome, lower back pain, and migraine headaches. Although these are very different forms of pain experience, similar mechanisms might be operating.

### Study 3: Juvenile rheumatoid arthritis

Chronic pain is a problem for children with juvenile rheumatoid arthritis. Anti-inflammatory agents used for their pain have ceiling effects, and other drugs such as narcotics cannot be used due to their addictive potential. Thus, massage therapy is being assessed for its usefulness for pain relief. In a study in which parents provided these children daily massages, several positive effects were noted (Field, Hernandez-Reif, Seligman et al 1997). The massaged children (versus the control children, who received progressive muscle relaxation) had:

1. decreased anxiety and cortisol after the first and last sessions
2. decreased pain over the 1-month period.

Juvenile rheumatoid arthritis (JRA) is the most common rheumatic disease of childhood and one of the most common chronic diseases of childhood (Cassidy & Petty 1995, Lovell & Walco 1989). The JRA diagnosis is based on the observation of persistent arthritis (6 or more weeks duration) in one or more joints. The disease typically manifests itself before 16 years of age, with peak onset in the age groups 1 to 3 and 8 to 12 years (Varni & Jay 1984). Common symptoms include night pain and joint stiffness both during the morning and following long periods of inactivity.

Treatment regimens for JRA have included medications, exercise and devices such as hand splints. The overall management of JRA consists of a multidisciplinary approach to comprehensive care, incorporating pharmacotherapy, physical and occupational therapy, orthopedic surgery, and psychosocial services. Despite the comprehensive approach to patient care, pain remains an undertreated clinical problem (Lovell & Walco 1989).

Because of the limited effects of anti-inflammatory drugs and the reluctance to use narcotics for pain reduction, investigators have been exploring other methods, including meditation, progressive muscle relaxation and guided imagery (Walco, Varni & Ilowite 1992). In the Walco et al (1992) study, 5- to 16-year-old children reported lower pain levels on visual analogue scales after eight sessions. In another study, modest pain reduction was achieved after training in progressive muscle relaxation, electromyogram (EMG) feedback, and thermal biofeedback (Lavigne et al 1992).

Children have also responded positively to massage as a relaxation therapy, but in a sample of children and adolescents who were stressed for reasons other than physical pain. For example, in one study, child and adolescent psychiatric patients given massage showed reduced depression, anxiety, and stress hormone levels (cortisol and norepinephrine), and their sleep increased (Field et al 1992). Increased sleep is frequently noted following massage, and it may contribute to the decreased pain noted in adult studies following massage. For example, in a study conducted on adults with fibromyalgia, increased sleep led to decreased pain (see study of this chapter), possibly because of less Substance P, which induces pain, being released during sleep. Although these possibilities are suggestive, the underlying mechanisms for massage therapy effects on pain are not yet known.

In our study on massage therapy with JRA children and adolescents the massages were expected to lower levels of anxiety, depression and pain as well as stress hormone (cortisol) levels. Teaching the parents to massage their children was also expected to give the parents a positive role in their child's treatment and thereby reduce their own anxiety levels.

## Method

**Subjects** Following the parents' informed consent and the children's assent, the sample was comprised of 20 children (14 females) age 5.4–14.8 years (mean = 9.8) who had been diagnosed with JRA on average 4.4 years previously and who were recruited from two rheumatologists. Entry criteria were (1) diagnosis of Juvenile Rheumatoid Arthritis by the pediatric rheumatologist, (2) age range between 4 and 16 years, and (3) no other serious or chronic illness. The mothers of 30 children identified as potential candidates for the study were approached at the time of a scheduled rheumatology clinic appointment. Two mothers refused to participate, six failed to return for follow-up assessments, and two moved out of the area. Thus, the final sample was comprised of 20 children. The children came from middle SES families (55% nuclear families) who were moderately educated (40% having at least some college education) and were distributed 40% White, 55% Hispanic, and 5% Black. Although as many as 65% of the mothers were employed, 90% were the children's primary caregivers. Ten percent of the parents and 25% of the children had previously received various kinds of massage therapy. On average the rheumatologists scored these children 7.4 on the Juvenile Arthritis Functional Assessment. This assessment was a modified form of the Activities of Daily Living Index developed by Walco et al (1992). This scale ranged from 0 to 46, with 0 being full functional activity and 46 being completely inactive. The physicians' average score of 7.4 suggested that the sample had mild functional limitations (dressing, bathing, eating, and gross motor activities). Children with severe limitations were excluded. The children were randomly assigned to massage therapy or relaxation therapy groups. The parents in each group were given live demonstrations and videotapes illustrating the therapy techniques. Typically, parents can learn this procedure after 30 minutes of demonstration and practice, and then they use the tape and daily practice to improve their skill. Having the parents, as opposed to massage therapists, massage their children empowers the parents for being part of their children's treatment process, reduces the parents' anxiety and stress hormone levels (recall the positive effects on the 'grandparent' volunteers in Chapter 1), and, of course, enables a more frequent and more cost-effective treatment for the children.

**Procedures**

*Standard medical care.* During the study the children continued to receive standard medical care including examinations by a pediatric rheumatologist.

*Massage therapy.* These children received a daily 15-minute massage by one of their parents for 30 days. This 15-minute massage was comprised of two standardized phases given in a progressive sequence typically followed by massage therapists. For the first phase, the child was placed in a supine position, and oil was applied to ensure smooth, continuous stroking movements. The parent stroked with some pressure the child's body in the following sequence:

1. *Face*:
    (a) strokes along both sides of the face
    (b) flats of fingers across the forehead
    (c) circular strokes over the temples and the hinge of the jaw
    (d) flat finger strokes over the nose, cheeks, jaw, and chin
2. *Stomach*:
    (a) hand-over-hand strokes in a paddlewheel fashion, avoiding the ribs and the tip of the rib cage
    (b) circular motion with fingers in a clockwise direction starting at the appendix
3. *Legs*:
    (a) strokes from hip to foot
    (b) squeezing and twisting in a wringing motion from hip to foot
    (c) massaging foot and toes
    (d) stretching the Achilles tendon
    (e) stroking the legs upward toward the heart
4. *Arms*:
    (a) stroking from the shoulders to the hands
    (b) same procedure as for the legs.

For the second phase, with the subject in a prone position, his or her back was massaged in the following sequence:

1. downward strokes along the back
2. hand-over-hand movements from the upper back to the buttocks
3. hands from side to side across the back, including the sides
4. circular motion from head to buttocks along, but not touching, the spine
5. simultaneous strokes over the sides of the back from the middle to the sides
6. rubbing and kneading shoulder muscles
7. rubbing the neck
8. stroking the length of the back
9. stroking from crown to feet.

The parent most involved with the child's medical regime was trained to administer the massage by a massage therapist who demonstrated it on the child. After the parent learned the procedure, the massage therapist watched the parent massaging the child. The parent was then given a written description of the massage as well as the videotaped demonstration and was asked to massage the child for 15 minutes at bedtime every day for 30 days.

*Relaxation therapy.* These children experienced a 15-minute relaxation session with their parents every night for 1 month. On the first day of the study, therapists trained and provided the parents with written instruction on the relaxation sessions. These sessions were performed with the subjects lying on their back and being instructed to tighten and flex different muscles of the body in a head to feet progression as was done in a study on children with psychiatric problems (Platania-Solazzo et al 1992). The following large muscle groups were involved: (1) face, (2) back, (3) arms, (4) hands, (5) thighs, (6) calves, and (7) feet. The parent was then given a written description of the relaxation session as well as the videotaped demonstration and was asked to conduct a relaxation session at bedtime every day for 30 days. Having a relaxation therapy control group enabled us to equate the children on amount of parental attention so that parental attention could be ruled out as an explanation for treatment group differences. Also, relaxation therapy has been somewhat effective for reducing anxiety and stress in children with various medical conditions. In order to adopt massage therapy as a standard treatment, it would need to be more effective than a less expensive treatment such as relaxation therapy.

**Assessments** A pediatric rheumatologist assessed the child's pain, and the parents completed questionnaires on their perception of their child's pain. Pain was also assessed by the child. Finally, a behaviour observation of the child's anxiety was made, and the child's saliva was assayed for stress hormone (cortisol) levels.

*Pre/post-session assessments.* Pre/post-session assessments were made before and after the sessions on the first and last days of the 30-day study, including:

- *STAI* (Spielberger et al 1970)
- *Behavior observation of the child's anxiety level*
- *Cortisol samples* (Appendix 2A).

*First-day/last-day assessments.* Parents' assessment of the child was made using the *Varni/Thompson Pediatric Pain Questionnaire* (PPQ) – *Parent Form* (Varni & Thompson 1985 unpublished, Varni, Thompson & Hanson 1987). The PPQ is administered within a structured interview format to assess the parents' perceptions of the child's pain prior to the child's physical examination by the pediatric rheumatologist. Pain is assessed on a visual analogue scale (VAS) (a 10 cm horizontal line with no number, marks, or descriptive vocabulary words along the length of the line but anchored by the phrases 'no pain' and 'severe pain'). The parent rates present pain and the worst pain for the previous week, pain severity at 9 a.m. and 9 p.m., and whether pain limited the child's school activity.

In addition to administering the parent version of the PPQ, parents were asked to answer how often the child's pain limited *vigorous* activities (e.g., running, bicycling, lifting heavy objects, or participating in strenuous sports), *moderate* activities (e.g., bending, walking several blocks, lifting, or stooping), and *mild* activities (e.g., walking one block, standing, sitting). Responses are made on a 6-point scale (0 = none of the time, 1 = 1 day only, 2 = 2–3 days, 3 = 4–7 days, 4 = more than one week, 5 = more than two weeks, and 6 = more than 3 weeks) designed to measure the frequency of the limitation. The total score, thus, has a range of 0 to 6, with optimal scores being lower.

In addition, the parents calculated the number of severe pain points the child was experiencing (on a drawing of the body). Using dorsal and frontal body diagrams, parents were asked to mark with an X the number of points where they believed the child was experiencing pain. Parents marked the most severe or painful points with a '1', moderately painful points were marked '2', and mildly painful points were marked '3'. A total score for severe pain points was derived by adding the number of points marked '1', with a lower number reflecting fewer severe points.

Child self-assessment was obtained using the *Varni/Thompson Pediatric Pain Questionnaire* (PPQ) – *Child Form* (Varni et al 1987). The PPQ can also be administered within a structured interview format to assess the children's perceptions of their pain. The child is interviewed by a researcher prior to his or her physical examination by the pediatric rheumatologist. Present pain and worst pain intensity for the previous week (pain past week) are assessed by a visual analogue scale (VAS). Each VAS is a 10 cm horizontal line with no numbers, marks, or descriptive vocabulary words along the length of the line. The child VAS is anchored with developmentally appropriate pain descriptors and happy and sad faces. A color-coded pain rating scale also measures pain intensity. Four developmentally appropriate categories of pain descriptors are provided along with eight standard crayons and a body outline.

The child is instructed to color in the four boxes underneath each descriptive category representing pain intensity, and then to color in the body outline with the selected color/intensity match to determine the number of severe pain points. In order to assess the sensory, affective and evaluative qualities of the child's pain experience, a list of pain descriptors is provided, with the child instructed to circle the words that most appropriately described his or her pain (words for child pain).

Physician assessment was made by the pediatric rheumatologist, who was blind to the child's group assignment and who assessed (1) the degree of pain, (2) the amount of morning stiffness (clinic was held during the mornings), and (3) the number of joints affected based on the physician's assessment. During the physical examination the child's pain level was also rated as severe, moderate, mild, quiescent (no physical or laboratory signs, on medication), or remission quiescent (2 months without medication). The joint was also rated as active based on evidence of inflammation, including calor (heat), dolor (pain), rubor (redness), or effusion (fluid). The pediatric rheumatologist completed this rating at the conclusion of the physical examination of the child.

## Results

Data analyses on the demographic characteristics of the two groups revealed no significant effects, suggesting the groups were similar at baseline.

**Pre/post-session assessments** Data analyses on the pre/post-session immediate effects revealed the following immediate effects favoring the massage group, including (see Table 2.6):

1. lower parent anxiety by self-report on the STAI
2. lower child anxiety based on behavioral observation
3. lower stress hormone levels (salivary cortisol) in the children receiving the massage.

**Table 2.6** Means for pre/post assessments for massage and relaxation group[1] (SDs in parentheses) (Study 3)

| Measures | Day 1 | | Day 30 | |
|---|---|---|---|---|
| | Pre | Post | Pre | Post |
| Parent anxiety (STAI) | 33.2 (11.0) | 27.0[1] (6.8) | 35.9 (11.5) | 34.3[1] (10.6) |
| | 30.5 (9.0) | 29.5 (7.1) | 30.7 (9.6) | 32.4 (8.9) |
| Child anxiety behavior[2] | 2.5 (0.7) | 3.0[1] (0.9) | 2.4 (0.5) | 2.9[1] (0.7) |
| | 2.6 (0.9) | 2.6 (0.7) | 2.5 (0.4) | 2.2 (0.4) |
| Child saliva cortisol (ng/mg)[3] | 1.5 (0.6) | 1.1[1] (0.4) | 1.1 (0.5) | 0.7[1] (0.6) |
| | 1.4 (0.4) | 1.5 (0.7) | 1.3 (0.4) | 1.1 (0.8) |

[1] Data for the relaxation group are in the lower row of each pair of rows.
[2] Higher score is optimal.
[3] Lower value is optimal.

### First-day/last-day assessments

*Child assessments of self.* Analyses of the child assessments of self on the first and last days revealed the following changes favoring the massage group (see Table 2.7):

1. fewer words for pain
2. less pain at present
3. less pain over the past week
4. fewer severe pain points.

*Parents' assessment of children.* Analyses of the first-day/last-day parent report measures revealed the following changes, by the last day, favoring the massaged children (see Table 2.8):

**Table 2.7**    Means for first-day/last-day massage and relaxation group[1] – child self-assessments (SDs in parentheses) (Study 3)

| Child self-assessment | First day | Last day |
|---|---|---|
| Words for pain | 14.1 (9.8) | 6.4** (4.1) |
| | 10.5 (7.6) | 12.0  (8.6) |
| Pain | | |
| present | 4.1 (1.9) | 1.1** (0.7) |
| | 4.9 (2.1) | 4.4  (2.1) |
| past week | 4.8 (2.0) | 1.6* (0.9) |
| | 3.5 (1.7) | 4.2  (2.0) |
| # severe pain points | 4.6 (2.3) | 1.6* (1.1) |
| | 4.9 (2.5) | 4.3  (2.4) |

[1] Data for the relaxation group are in the lower row of each pair of rows.
* $p < 0.05$; ** $p < 0.005$.

**Table 2.8**    Means for first-day/last-day massage and relaxation group[1] – parent assessments (SDs in parentheses) (Study 3)

| Parent assessment of child | First day | Last day |
|---|---|---|
| Pain | | |
| present | 2.9 (1.7) | 0.7  (0.4) |
| | 3.4 (2.1) | 3.5  (2.0) |
| past week | 6.9 (3.8) | 1.7**** (1.2) |
| | 6.8 (3.1) | 6.2  (4.3) |
| # severe pain points | 6.0 (4.2) | 4.1* (2.4) |
| | 8.2 (4.7) | 6.4  (3.7) |
| severity at 9 a.m. | 4.0 (3.0) | 4.9  (3.0) |
| | 6.0 (4.7) | 5.0  (3.9) |
| severity at 9 p.m. | 4.0 (2.2) | 1.0** (0.4) |
| | 5.2 (2.9) | 6.0  (3.2) |
| Pain limiting activities | | |
| School activity | 2.3 (1.4) | 2.0  (1.4) |
| | 2.8 (1.9) | 2.4  (1.0) |
| Vigorous activity | 4.2 (2.1) | 1.9*** (0.7) |
| | 4.6 (2.4) | 4.1  (2.9) |

[1] Data for the relaxation group are in the lower row of each pair of rows.
* $p < 0.05$; ** $p < 0.01$; *** $p < 0.005$; **** $p < 0.001$.

1. less pain at present
2. less pain over the past week
3. fewer severe pain points
4. less pain severity at 9 p.m. in the evening
5. less pain limiting of vigorous activity.

*Physician's assessment of children.* Analyses of the first-day/last-day physician's assessment revealed the following changes favoring the massaged children (see Table 2.9):

1. less pain
2. less morning stiffness.

## Discussion

The immediate effects of the massage therapy, including the reduced anxiety levels in the parents administering the massage, lower child anxiety based on behavioral observations, and lower stress hormone (salivary cortisol) levels in the children, were perhaps not surprising, because other studies on massage therapy with children have reported similar effects. For example, studies on diabetic and asthmatic children (Field, Hernandez-Reif, LaGreca et al 1997, Field, Henteleff et al 1998), and child psychiatric patients (Field et al 1992) have also revealed the immediate anxiety-alleviating and stress-hormone-reducing effects of massage therapy.

The longer-term effects bear on the pain-alleviating properties of massage therapy. Several measures based on assessments made by the children and parents converged to suggest less pain during the present and past weeks and fewer severe pain points. The children also provided fewer words for pain, which has been a reliable measure in other studies on JRA (Varni & Bernstein 1991). Additional measures completed by the parents also suggested less severe pain during the evening (9 p.m.) and less pain limiting

**Table 2.9** Means for first-day/last-day massage and relaxation group[1] – physician assessment (SDs in parentheses) (Study 3)

| Physician assessment | First day | Last day |
|---|---|---|
| Degree of pain | 30.0 (19.2) | 14.1* (10.8) |
|  | 29.2 (16.4) | 20.8 (12.3) |
| Morning stiffness (min) | 5.7 (2.7) | 1.2* (0.8) |
|  | 1.7 (0.9) | 4.2 (2.1) |
| # of joints | 2.2 (1.6) | 1.7 (0.9) |
|  | 2.6 (1.2) | 2.5 (1.3) |

[1] Data for the relaxation group are in the lower row of each pair of rows.
* $p < 0.05$.

of vigorous activity. Finally, the physician's assessment provided confirmatory data suggesting less pain and less morning stiffness by the end of the month of massage therapy.

These pain-alleviating effects may derive from simple relaxation and anxiety-reducing effects of massage therapy as has been reported in other studies on the use of relaxation therapy with children experiencing JRA (Lavigne et al 1992, Varni & Jay 1984) and other studies on the use of massage therapy with children experiencing other medical conditions (Field 1995). Direction of causality, i.e. whether reduced anxiety and stress hormones leads to reduced pain or reduced pain leads to less anxiety and lower stress hormones, is impossible to know from this study. Parent and child anxiety have been known to at least exacerbate painful medical conditions (Fries, Spitz & Young 1982).

The results of this study parallel those noted in a recent study on the use of massage therapy with adults diagnosed with fibromyalgia (Sunshine et al 1996). Two possible interpretations were offered for those data, including the gate theory – i.e. pressure receptors are longer and more myelinated than pain fibers and therefore the pressure stimuli are transmitted faster, closing the gate to pain signals (Melzack & Wall 1965). Another more recent theory is that massage therapy increases restorative (deep or quiet) sleep, and thus less Substance P (pain transmitter) is released (Sunshine et al 1996). Future studies might record sleep patterns to assess this potential mechanism as well as other possible explanatory measures.

In summary, this study suggests that parents massaging their children with JRA before bedtime each night can help decrease their anxiety and stress hormone levels. After 30 days of massage therapy, the children were also experiencing less pain, thus confirming the pain-relieving effects of massage therapy. Although the underlying mechanism for the relationship between massage therapy and pain reduction is not known, massage seems to be a cost-effective therapy for children with juvenile rheumatoid arthritis. The parents reported that they enjoyed massaging their children and felt that they were 'contributing to their treatment'. Massage therapy may have been more effective than relaxation therapy because the children may have been too young to understand and actively participate in the relaxation therapy. Further research is needed to compare the relative efficacy and the costs and benefits of these therapies in different age groups, as well as any long-term effects. Finally, studies are needed on the underlying mechanisms that might explain the pain-reducing effects of massage therapy.

## Study 4: Fibromyalgia

In a study on fibromyalgia syndrome (pain all over the body for no known etiology), participants were randomly assigned to one of three conditions:

1. massage therapy
2. transcutaneous electrical stimulation (TENS), a steel roller the size of a pen that transmits a small, barely discernible current as it is rolled across the body
3. transcutaneous electrical stimulation without current (sham TENS)

for 30-minute treatment sessions two times per week for 5 weeks (Sunshine et al 1996). The massage therapy subjects reported lower anxiety and depression, and their cortisol levels were lower immediately after the therapy sessions on the first and last days of the study. The massage therapy group improved on a dolorimeter measure of pain, reported less pain, less stiffness and fatigue and fewer nights of difficult sleeping. Thus, massage therapy was the most effective therapy with these fibromyalgia patients.

Fibromyalgia was once considered a depressive disorder. However, this view has been replaced by the new theory that both central and peripheral pain mechanisms are activated in these patients. For example, disturbances in muscle microcirculation have been reported (Bartels & Danneskiold-Samse 1986, Bengtsson, Henriksson & Larsson 1986, Simms 1994), as well as alterations in restorative sleep and neuroendocrine function, resulting in low levels of serotonin, growth hormone, and somatomedin-C (Bennett 1993). In addition, Substance P levels in the cerebrospinal fluid are significantly elevated in this patient population (Russell et al 1993, Vaeroy et al 1988).

Fibromyalgia patients tend to have multiple symptoms including generalized pain, myalgia, arthralgia, nonrestorative sleep, irritable bowel, temporomandibular dysfunction, anxiety, depression, headache, and neuropsychiatric complaints. Unfortunately, many traditional therapies, both pharmacological and nonpharmacological, have yielded little or no benefit. Although many nonmedicinal treatments have been proposed, few controlled studies of this type have been published (McCain 1989, Yunus & Masi 1985).

Fibromyalgia syndrome (FMS) patients may benefit from massage therapy because it enhances immunological and neuroendocrine function: for example, decreasing cortisol and norepinephrine levels and increasing serotonin levels and natural killer cell activity. The low serotonin levels in fibromyalgia patients have been related to their nonrestorative sleep, mood alteration, and increased pain sensitivity. In at least one study, massage therapy increased serotonin levels (Ironson et al 1996), and in another, sleep patterns improved (Field et al 1992). Although these data are suggestive, they are based on studies with other disease groups.

The purpose of the present study was to determine the effects of massage therapy on pain, depression and anxiety associated with fibromyalgia. Massage therapy was compared with microcurrent transcutaneous electrical stimulation (TENS) as another possible therapy. This was performed in a double blind fashion using sham TENS as a control.

## Method

**Subjects** Thirty female adult FMS patients were recruited from local rheumatology practices. These patients were not receiving any other treatment at the time of the study. They averaged 49.8 years (range = 18–80), were middle income levels on average, and were distributed 32% Caucasian, 44% Hispanic, and 24% Black. The subjects were randomly assigned (using a table of random numbers) to one of three groups, massage therapy, TENS, and sham TENS. The three groups of women did not differ on the demographic variables of ethnicity, income, or age. The physician and researchers responsible for the pre and post assessments were 'blind' to the group assignment of the subjects. Assessments were made only during the first and last sessions (session 1 and session 10).

**Procedure** Before the study period the subjects were assessed by a rheumatologist to determine the fibromyalgia diagnosis according to the criteria established by the American College of Rheumatology. Point pressure threshold was measured with the use of a dolorimeter by exerting a force of 1 kg/s over the 18 tender points outlined in the ACR classification criteria. All pre and post tests were performed by the same rheumatologist (WS, the primary author). A global rating of pain was also recorded by the rheumatologist on the first and last days of therapy. Patients were required to maintain their pharmacological regimen during the course of the study.

The *immediate effects* of these therapies were measured by the *State Trait Anxiety Inventory (STAI)* (Spielberger et al 1970), the Profile of Mood States (McNair et al 1971), which measures the subjects' feelings of depressed mood at the moment, and by stress hormone (salivary cortisol) levels (Radloff 1977). The *end of study effects* (end of the study versus beginning of the study period) were assessed by the dolorimeter test, an interview on pain, sleep, and daily functioning, and by the CES–D (depression scale) (Radloff 1977).

*Massage therapy.* The massage therapy sessions consisted of moderate pressure stroking of the head, neck, shoulders, back, arms, hands, legs, and feet for 30 minutes.

*TENS and sham TENS.* The TENS and sham TENS groups received tactile stimulation with the TENS roller, in the latter case with no current. The microcurrent TENS stimulator, the Electro-Acuscope is a metal rod that delivers electrical stimulation that is not strong enough to cause muscular contraction or perceived skin irritation, and the subject cannot feel the electrical stimulation. What the subject feels is simply the mechanical stroking of the rod-like metallic moveable surface electrodes. The therapist moves the rod over the patient's body (the same body parts that were massaged in that group). The dials and knobs of the transmitting equipment were hidden from view of the therapist and the subject, blinding both of them to the protocol. For those receiving sham TENS the Electro-Acuscope was never turned on. Neither the therapist nor the subject knew whether electrical stimulation was being delivered. However, the therapist still rolled the rod on the subject in both of these groups which means that a form of tactile stimulation was received by all three groups. The two TENS groups were informed that they would not be told their group assignment until the completion of the study. Although the TENS and sham TENS groups were double blind, there was no way, of course, to double blind the massage therapy group.

## Results

**Pre/post-therapy immediate effects measures** Analyses of the immediate effects measures revealed the following:

1. The massage therapy group had lower State Anxiety (STAI), lower depressed mood (POMS) scores, and lower salivary cortisol levels after therapy versus before therapy on the first and last sessions (see Table 2.10)

2. The TENS group had lower State Anxiety and depressed mood scores and lower salivary cortisol levels after therapy but only on the last session (see Table 2.11)

3. No changes were noted for the sham TENS group (see Table 2.12).

**Table 2.10**  Means for massage therapy group (Study 4)

|  | First session | | Last session | |
|---|---|---|---|---|
| Variables[1] | Pre | Post | Pre | Post |
| *Pre/post-therapy* | | | | |
| Anxiety (STAI) | 45.4 | 35.0**** | 38.6 | 34.1* |
| Depression (POMS) | 17.3 | 12.9* | 21.3 | 12.0* |
| Stress hormone (ng cortisol) | 1.9 | 1.2* | 1.8 | 1.0* |
| *First-day/last-day* | **First session** | | **Last session** | |
| *Physician's assessment* | | | | |
| Rating of clinical condition (0–10) | 4.3 | | 1.8* | |
| Dolorimeter value (kg) | 3.4 | | 4.5** | |
| *Self-report* | | | | |
| *Pain and sleep symptoms* | | | | |
| Pain | 8.6 | | 5.3**** | |
| Pain last week | 7.8 | | 6.0** | |
| Stiffness | 8.6 | | 6.8** | |
| Fatigue | 7.4 | | 4.5** | |
| # Nights difficult sleeping | 6.1 | | 3.4*** | |
| *Depression scale (CES–D)* | 31.9 | | 26.8 | |

[1] All variables are ratings except where otherwise specified.
* $p = 0.05$; ** $p = 0.01$; *** $p = 0.005$; **** $p = 0.001$ for adjacent values.

**Table 2.11**  Means for transcutaneous electrical stimulation group (Study 4)

|  | First session | | Last session | |
|---|---|---|---|---|
| Variables[1] | Pre | Post | Pre | Post |
| *Pre/post-therapy* | | | | |
| Anxiety (STAI) | 45.2 | 37.3 | 43.1 | 33.0** |
| Depression (POMS) | 15.5 | 12.7 | 19.6 | 11.8** |
| Stress hormone (ng cortisol) | 2.1 | 1.5 | 1.9 | 1.5* |
| *First-day/last-day* | **First session** | | **Last session** | |
| *Physician's assessment* | | | | |
| Rating of clinical condition (0–10) | 6.1 | | 3.8** | |
| Dolorimeter value (kg) | 0.8 | | 3.2 | |
| *Self-report* | | | | |
| *Pain and sleep symptoms* | | | | |
| Pain | 7.5 | | 7.3 | |
| Pain last week | 7.9 | | 6.7 | |
| Stiffness | 7.2 | | 7.1 | |
| Fatigue | 7.6 | | 7.1 | |
| #Nights difficult sleeping | 4.0 | | 4.2 | |
| *Depression scale (CES–D)* | 34.3 | | 27.8 | |

[1] All variables are ratings except where otherwise specified.
* $p = 0.05$, ** $p = 0.01$ for adjacent values.

**Table 2.12** Means for sham transcutaneous electrical stimulation group (Study 4)

| Variables[1] | First session | | Last session | |
|---|---|---|---|---|
| | Pre | Post | Pre | Post |
| *Pre/post-therapy* | | | | |
| Anxiety (STAI) | 49.2 | 40.0 | 42.6 | 37.6 |
| Depression (POMS) | 19.0 | 17.4 | 11.7 | 13.7 |
| Stress hormone (ng cortisol) | 1.7 | 1.4 | 1.6 | 1.6 |
| *First-day/last-day* | **First session** | | **Last session** | |
| *Physician's assessment* | | | | |
| Rating of clinical condition (0–10) | 4.8 | | 3.2** | |
| Dolorimeter value (kg) | 2.9 | | 3.5 | |
| *Self-report* | | | | |
| *Pain and sleep symptoms* | | | | |
| Pain | 8.8 | | 7.2 | |
| Pain last week | 8.0 | | 5.9 | |
| Stiffness | 7.8 | | 6.5** | |
| Fatigue | 8.7 | | 6.9 | |
| Nights difficult sleeping | 5.3 | | 4.0 | |
| *Depression scale (CES–D)* | 29.3 | | 29.4 | |

[1] All variables are ratings except where otherwise specified.
* $p = 0.05$, ** $p = 0.01$ for adjacent values.

**First-session/last-session measures (longer-term effects)** Analyses of the longer-term measures suggested the following.

1. The massage therapy group improved on the rheumatologist's rating of clinical condition and dolorimeter value, and those subjects reported fewer symptoms at the end of the study, including less pain, less pain over the last week, less stiffness, less fatigue, and fewer nights of difficult sleeping.

2. The TENS group only improved on the physician's assessment of clinical condition.

3. The sham TENS group also improved on the physician's assessment of clinical condition but less than did the other two groups.

## Discussion

A step effect occurred, with the massage therapy being more effective than TENS, which in turn was more effective than sham TENS stimulation in decreasing anxiety and depression. Although both the massage therapy and TENS groups reported lower anxiety and depressed mood, and although they had lower salivary cortisol levels following the therapy sessions on the last day, only the massage therapy group showed those changes on both the first and last days.

The rheumatologist's assessment of the subjects' clinical condition improved for all three groups. This suggests that all three forms of tactile stimulation and attention were somewhat effective, including sham TENS (which was also a form of tactile stimulation). However, only the massage therapy group improved on the dolorimeter and the subjects' self-reports of pain.

Further support for the superiority of the massage therapy is suggested by those subjects reporting fewer symptoms by the end of the study, including less pain, stiffness, fatigue, and difficulty sleeping. Since the subjects' symptoms are the primary target of treatment, it is noteworthy that improvement occurred particularly for those symptoms that are most frequently reported among FMS subjects.

The most effective aspect of massage therapy is not clear. For example, the psychological effects of hands-on treatment may be uniquely important. The subjects in the massage therapy group may have felt that they were receiving more attention. As in other forms of therapy, it is not clear how long the benefits persist. Patients may need a steady dose of the massage therapy for continuous alleviation of pain. Future research will need to assess the long-term benefits.

## Study 5: Premenstrual syndrome

Premenstrual syndrome (PMS) has been described as a complex of symptoms recurring at a specific time every month (Keenan et al 1992, Rivera-Tovar, Pilknois & Frank 1992). Women have reported over 150 complaints related to PMS, including irritability, depression, lethargy, poor coordination, swelling of the abdomen and extremities, breast discomfort, headaches, weight gain, and fluid retention (Freeman et al 1996, Stout & Steege 1985). In adolescent women, PMS has been linked to poor academic performance (Boyle 1997) and in working women to lower job performance (High & Marcellino 1995). Women who suffer from PMS also report encountering more stressful occurrences during the premenstrual period (Fontana & Badawy 1997).

Treatments for PMS range from psychotropic medications for depressive symptoms (Freeman et al 1996, Steiner 1996) to hormonal therapy (Morse et al 1991, Steiner 1996) to surgical interventions, such as hysterectomy for severe cases (Metcalf 1995). Although antidepressant medications appear to effectively treat PMS (Sundblad et al 1992, Wood et al 1992), side effects such as insomnia, nausea, headache and gastrointestinal upset lead some women to discontinue the medication (Freeman et al 1996).

Women with PMS often self-prescribe over-the-counter analgesics for pain relief. Use of analgesics beyond the premenstrual phase has been documented among women with PMS, increasing the probability of pain medication abuse (Hart & Hill 1997).

Alternative therapies for PMS have been recommended and have included nutritional supplements such as vitamins and oils (Corney & Stanton 1991) and diuretics to control salt and water balance (Rausch & Parry 1993). Coping skills training and relaxation therapy have been somewhat effective for treating symptoms associated with PMS (Morse et al 1991). One study reported attenuated PMS symptoms with relaxation therapies, combined with behavioral treatment, diet, and exercise (Pearlstein et al 1992). In that study, however, the simple effects of relaxation therapy on PMS could not be determined, because of the multiple treatment design. Also the effects usually wear off after a few menstrual cycles, thus forcing women to seek alternative treatments (Rubinow & Roy-Byrne 1984).

Massage therapy has not been explored for PMS, although current research suggests it is effective for reducing stress, anxiety, and depression and alleviating pain. For example, massage therapy has been found to reduce depressive symptoms and related stress hormones (cortisol) in depressed teenage mothers (Field, Grizzle, Scafidi & Schanberg 1996) and in depressed and anxious psychiatric adolescents (Field et al 1992). Massage therapy has also been effective in reducing the generalized pain of fibromyalgia (Sunshine et al 1996) and ameliorating fatigue-related symptoms, particularly emotional stress and somatic symptoms, associated with chronic fatigue syndrome (Field, Sunshine et al 1997). Also, significant pain reduction has been reported from massage therapy for lower back pain (Hernandez-Reif et al 1999) and migraine (Hernandez-Reif et al 1998).

The present study measured massage therapy versus relaxation effects on women with premenstrual syndrome. Although relaxation therapy was expected to decrease anxious symptoms, the women receiving massage therapy were expected to report lower anxiety, depression, and pain and a reduction of PMS symptoms during the week prior to the onset of menstruation.

## Method

**Subjects** Twenty-four women between the ages of 19 and 45 (mean age = 33 years) who fulfilled the following criteria were recruited from gynecological practices:

1. premenstrual discomfort for at least 6 months

2. not currently taking birth control pills, hormonal, or psychotropic medications
3. not taking any medication throughout the study
4. menstrual cycles lasting between 24 and 30 days
5. duration of menstruation not longer than 7 days
6. not pregnant or lactating for the 6 months prior
7. premenstrual symptoms ending at the onset of menses
8. score greater than a 20 point difference on the menstrual distress questionnaire (Moos 1968), when first administered during the follicular phase and later in the late luteal phase. Subjects were predominantly middle socioeconomic status (mean = 2.2 on Hollingshead Two Factor Index). Ethnically, the women were distributed 38% Caucasian, 46% Hispanic, 8% African American, and 8% other. They were randomly assigned to a massage or relaxation therapy group based on a stratification procedure to ensure homogeneity for age and severity of symptoms. There were no initial group differences on demographic or symptom severity variables.

**Procedures** After initial contact, and meeting inclusion criteria, the subjects were randomly assigned to a massage therapy or a relaxation group.

*Massage therapy.* The massage group subjects received a 30-minute massage, twice per week for 5 weeks (10 massages), beginning during their premenstrual week (in order to establish the baseline measures), and ending on the last day of their premenstrual week of the following cycle. For the first 15 minutes, with the participant facing up, the massage consisted of:

1. stroking and kneading of the muscles in the neck
2. outward stroking on the forehead towards the temple and to the jaw
3. pressing down on the tops of the shoulder
4. pressure to mid-shoulder trigger points (tender points)
5. long gliding stroking to the hand, arm, and shoulder area
6. circular stroking on the stomach and gentle lifting of soft tissue over the stomach area, followed by
7. stroking the feet, stroking the leg (from the foot to the hip) and kneading of thigh muscles.

For the last 15 minutes, with the participant facing down, the massage consisted of

1. stretching the ankle and Achilles tendon
2. squeezing and compressing calf muscles
3. kneading the muscles of the thigh

4. long gliding stroking of the leg (from the heel up and over the hip)
5. gentle pressing into the low back and stroking toward the sides of the body
6. parallel stroking to the spine up to the shoulders and out to the arms
7. squeezing the top of the shoulders
8. squeezing the soft tissue on the back of the neck
9. long stroking from the shoulders down the entire back surface of the body to the toes.

*Relaxation therapy.* Rather than a standard control group, a progressive muscle relaxation therapy procedure was used in this study to control for placebo effects. A therapist provided subjects with written instructions and training on how to tense and relax major muscle groups. Following the training session, subjects were instructed to perform 30 minutes of progressive muscle relaxation sessions twice a week on the same schedule as the massage therapy group. These relaxation sessions consisted of tensing and relaxing large muscle groups, starting with the feet and progressing to the calves, legs, hands, arms, back, and face.

**Assessments** Assessments were completed during the week prior to the onset of menstruation. Before the massage and relaxation sessions on the first and last day of the study, self-rating scales were given, including the Menstrual Distress Questionnaire, *State Trait Anxiety Inventory (STAI)*, the Profile of Mood States, and a Visual Analogue Scale on perceived pain intensity. Immediately after the massage or relaxation session, the *State Trait Anxiety Inventory (STAI)*, Profile of Mood States, and Visual Analogue Scales on pain were again completed.

*Pre/post-session (immediate effects).* The immediate effects were measured by the *State Trait Anxiety Inventory* (STAI) (Spielberger et al 1970), the *Profile of Moods States* (POMS) (McNair et al 1971), and the *Visual Analogue Scale* (VAS) of the PPQ.

*First-day/last-day measures (longer-term effects).* Longer-term effects were measured by the *Menstrual Distress Questionnaire* (MDQ) (Moos 1968). This is a 47-item scale including eight subgroups of symptoms that are rated on a six-point scale ranging from not at all to partially disabling. The subgroups are pain (e.g., headaches, cramps, backache), concentration (e.g., forgetfulness, confusion, distractibility), behavioral change (e.g., lowered school or job performance, avoidance of social activities, staying at home), autonomic reactions (e.g., faint, cold sweats, vomiting), water retention (e.g., weight gain, skin disorders, swelling), negative affect (e.g., crying, loneliness, depression), arousal (e.g., orderliness, bursts of energy, excitement), and control (e.g., heart pounding, feeling of suffocation, fuzzy vision). In addition to the eight subgroup scores, the questionnaire yields a total symptom distress score. The questionnaire has adequate internal consistency and construct validity (Moos 1968, Coppen & Kessel 1963). Subjects in the massage therapy group were expected to report lower symptom severity following treatment.

## Results

Analyses of the immediate-effects variables (see Table 2.13) revealed:

1. decreased anxiety levels for the massage group on the first and last day of the study and only on the first day for the relaxation group
2. improved mood for the massage group after the first and last massage sessions
3. a reduction in pain for the massage group after the first and last massage sessions

**Table 2.13** Means for massage and relaxation groups for pre/post-therapy (Study 5)

| | Massage | | Relaxation | |
|---|---|---|---|---|
| First/Last-day measures | First day | Last day | First day | Last day |
| | Pre/post | Pre/post | Pre/post | Pre/post |
| *Short-term measures* | | | | |
| STAI (anxiety) | 54.5/33.9**** | 48.9/24.7*** | 51.6/35.3**** | 51.5/41.4 |
| POMS (mood) | 18.4/ 4.0**** | 14.9/ 1.1** | 17.1/10.0 | 16.6/11.6 |
| VAS (pain) | 2.3/ 0.5**** | 1.5/ 0.1*** | 2.8/ 1.9 | 2.6/ 1.7 |
| *Longer term measures* | | | | |
| CES-D (depression) | 24.0 | 20.5 | 25.7 | 24.0 |
| MDQ (menstrual distress) | 98.2 | 76.8* | 90.2 | 87.0 |
| Pain | 17.5 | 11.8** | 14.8 | 13.6 |
| Concentration | 16.8 | 14.2 | 15.0 | 15.8 |
| Behavioral change | 11.4 | 9.0 | 10.4 | 10.5 |
| Autonomic reaction | 6.4 | 5.1 | 6.1 | 5.9 |
| Water retention | 9.6 | 7.3** | 8.5 | 8.8 |
| Negative affect | 20.3 | 14.7 | 18.4 | 16.6 |
| Arousal | 8.0 | 8.3 | 8.2 | 7.6 |
| Control | 8.3 | 6.5 | 8.8 | 8.2 |

Asterisks indicate significance level for adjacent numbers: * $p < 0.05$; ** $p < 0.01$; *** $p < 0.005$; **** $p < 0.001$.

Analyses of the longer-term-effects variables (Table 2.13) revealed:

1. an improvement in the overall PMS symptom profile for the massage group
2. a reduction in pain
3. a reduction in water retention for the massage group by the last day of the study.

### Discussion

The data reflected an immediate decrease in anxiety for the PMS women after the first massage and the first relaxation session. Anxiety also decreased after the last day session, but only for the massage group. These data are consistent with other massage therapy studies documenting decreased anxiety for other pain syndromes and painful conditions, including childbirth labor pain (Field, Hernandez-Reif, Taylor et al 1997), fibromyalgia (Sunshine et al 1996), and debridement procedures (skin brushing) for burn patients (Field, Peck et al 1998).

The marked improvement in mood for the women in the massage group is of particular clinical importance because depressed mood is a major symptom of PMS (Steiner 1996). Depressed mood has also been noted to disrupt or interfere with job and academic productivity and social activity in these women (High & Marcellino 1995). The improved mood following massage therapy was not surprising, as it has also improved after massage therapy for other pain syndromes and chronic conditions, including chronic fatigue syndrome (Field, Sunshine et al 1997), post-traumatic stress disorder (Field, Seligman et al 1996) and HIV (Ironson et al 1996).

The decreased pain scores on two scales (the VAS and the pain scale on the Menstrual Distress Questionnaire) are consistent with the pain reduction noted in other massage research on painful conditions, including fibromyalgia (Sunshine et al 1996) and childbirth labor pain (Field, Hernandez-Reif, Taylor et al 1997). Further support for the therapeutic value of massage for PMS is provided by the reduction in water retention reported by the women, the most commonly reported symptom along with pain during the premenstrual period.

Future research in this area is needed to determine whether continued massage sessions lead to continued improvement in PMS symptoms. In addition, outcome parameters that include job or academic absenteeism and a measure of social activity and relationship functioning would be informative.

## Study 6: Migraine headaches

Alternative therapies for chronic headaches are currently under study. Treatments such as relaxation, biofeedback, hypnosis, and exercise are attractive to people because they do not have the side effects associated with pharmacotherapy (e.g., dizziness, nausea, sleeplessness, kidney or liver disease, toxicity (Van Der Meer 1990). The few studies that exist on alternative therapies have mixed results. For example, while some have reported that individuals with headaches can benefit from relaxation training by decreasing peak headache intensity and increasing the number of headache-free days (Andrasik et al 1984), others report that relaxation therapy has little effect on pain reduction (Cott et al 1992, Gauthier, Ivers & Carrier 1996). In contrast, biofeedback-assisted relaxation has been successful in decreasing pain and medication intake in addition to possibly influencing vasodilation (McGrady et al 1994, Wauquier et al 1995). Although hypnosis has been shown to reduce self-reported headache pain, it did not decrease the need for analgesics (ter Kuile et al 1995). Exercise (Darling 1991, Lockett & Campbell 1990) and physical therapy (Hickling, Silverman & Loos 1990, Jensen, Nielsen & Vosmar 1990) have been somewhat effective in reducing chronic headaches. Cervical spine manipulation has also been used to treat head and neck pain (for a review, see Vernon 1995). However, this treatment can be dangerous and has been associated with brain stem dysfunction (Mueller & Sahs 1976, O'Neill 1994).

Massage therapy has reduced anxiety and stress hormones, including cortisol and norepinephrine (Field et al 1992), has increased serotonin levels (5-HIAA) (Field, Grizzle, Scafidi, Abrams & Richardson 1996), has decreased pain associated with other pain conditions such as fibromyalgia (Sunshine et al 1996), juvenile rheumatoid arthritis (Field, Hernandez-Reif et al 1997) and chronic lower back pain (Hernandez-Reif, Field, Krasnegor et al 1999), and has reduced sleep disturbances (Field et al 1992, Field & Hernandez-Reif 1998).

Although several studies have also suggested that massage therapy reduces headaches, many of these have methodological problems. For example, Lipton (1986) found that vigorous compression and massage to the head at the onset of a migraine reduces headaches. However, the study was methodologically flawed because it lacked a control group, the length of the massage and techniques were not controlled, and no statistical analyses were reported. Other investigations reporting positive effects of manual therapy for post-traumatic headache (Jensen et al 1990) and/or physical therapy for chronic tension headache (Hammill, Cook & Rosecrance 1996, Puustjarvi, Aoraksinen & Pontinen 1990) also lacked control groups. In another study, a combination of massage with various forms of Eastern therapies, including acupuncture, for example, reduced headaches (Meyer 1993). However, the massage therapy effects were clearly confounded by the other treatments.

The present study used a control group, had several therapists administer a standardized massage therapy protocol, and assessed psychological as well as biochemical effects. Serotonin has been implicated in the etiology of muscle contraction and vascular headaches (Marcus 1993), and massage therapy has been noted to increase serotonin levels (Field et al 1996). Based on our studies with other pain syndromes, massage therapy was expected to (1) reduce anxiety, (2) reduce stress hormones (salivary cortisol and urinary catecholamine levels), (3) increase serotonin levels, (4) reduce the frequency and severity of headaches, (5) decrease medication intake, and (6) decrease sleep disturbances.

## Method

**Participants** The sample included 26 adults (22 women) ranging in age from 24 to 65 (mean = 39.9; SD = 8.8). They were middle socioeconomic status (Hollingshead Index mean = 2.3) and were distributed 69% Caucasian, 27% Hispanic, and 4% African American. The inclusion criterion was chronic headaches for a period of at least 6 months (mean = 20.7 years). Nineteen participants were diagnosed with migraine without aura (a warming sensation), three with migraine with aura, two with migraine with aura plus chronic tension-type headache, and two with migraine without aura plus chronic tension-type headache. Fourteen participants reported one or more family members having a chronic headache condition. Participants were assigned to a massage therapy or a control group. No differences were found between groups on demographic variables (i.e., age, ethnicity, sex, and socioeconomic status) or headache type.

**Procedures**

*Standard medical care.* During the study period, both the control and massage groups continued their medication regimen. The massage and the control groups did not differ on baseline medication intake.

*Massage therapy.* The 30-minute massage sessions were given twice a week for 5 consecutive weeks by trained massage therapists. With the participant in a supine position, the therapist started by applying pressure, circular friction and kneading to the muscles on the back of the neck, followed by

1. two-fingered, semicircular stroking to the base of the skull
2. palpating under the base of the skull
3. head and neck mobilization while using thumb to apply compression to suboccipital fibers
4. steady, rhythmic pressure to the groove along the base of the skull (see King 1995 for a more detailed description of techniques). This 10-minute routine was repeated three times for the 30-minute sessions.

**Assessments** Both groups were assessed on the first day and again 5 weeks later on the last day of the study. Pre/post-session assessments were administered before and after the massage or control period and provided immediate-effects data. The first/ last day measures were assessed before the treatment or control period and provided longer-term effects of the treatment.

*Medical and headache history questionnaires* (Appendix 2B). These were administered for the purpose of diagnosing the headache condition according to the headache classifications established by the International Headache Society (Saper et al 1995). Questions for diagnosing headache type included descriptors for headache pain (e.g., nagging, throbbing, stabbing), headache severity (i.e., mild, moderate, severe, or incapacitating), frequency (by days), duration (by hours), location of pain (e.g., unilateral, bilateral, bandlike around the head, occipital), and symptoms, if any, associated with headache (e.g., vomiting, nausea, tearing of eye, swelling of eyelid on side of pain, aversion to light, noise, odor). Final diagnostic decisions were made by a board-certified physician specializing in chronic headaches (Dr Swerdlow).

*Pre/post session measures (immediate effects).* These included:

1. the *Vitas Pain Scale*. (Vitas Health Care Corporation 1993 unpublished). Present headache pain intensity was assessed with a visual analogue scale ranging from 0 (no pain) to 10 (worst pain) and anchored with five faces. The faces, located at two point intervals, ranged from very happy (0), to happy (2), contented (4), somewhat distressed (6), distressed (8), to very distressed (10)
2. *Saliva sample* (Appendix 2A) for cortisol.

*First/last day session measures (longer-term effects).* These included the following.

1. The *Symptom Checklist-90-R* (SCL-90-R) (Derogatis 1983). This checklist was administered to assess depression, anxiety, hostility, and somatization symptoms typically associated with

chronic headaches (Dieter & Swerdlow 1988). Items on the four different dimensions reflected distress experienced over the past week and were rated on a 5-point scale ranging from 0 (not at all) to 4 (extremely).

2. The *Headache Log*. Headache frequency and intensity were assessed with the Headache Log (Dieter & Swerdlow 1988, Swerdlow & Dieter 1989). Using a calendar diary, participants rated their most intense headache of the day on a four-point scale with 0 = no head pain, 1 = mild (irritating pain), 2 = moderate (interfering pain), and 3 = severe (incapacitating pain). Dividing the sum of the days that a participant experienced each headache intensity by the total number of monitored days provided the Percentage of Days Score (PDS) for each type of headache pain (i.e., mild, moderate, severe). A Global Headache Score (GHS) was calculated by first calculating the number of days at each headache intensity, then multiplying the number of days by the corresponding intensity value (i.e., 1,2,3) and then adding these three scores and dividing by the number of monitored days. Higher values reflected a more severe headache condition.

3. The *Medication Log*. The types of analgesic medications taken during the previous month (baseline/first day) and during the 5-week study period (treatment/last day) were recorded and averaged across participants in each group. The massage group was expected to report a reduction in analgesic intake.

4. The *Sleep Diary*. Participants logged the number of hours they slept and the number of nightwakings for the previous night on a daily calendar. The massage group subjects were expected to report fewer sleep disturbances (Field et al 1992, Field & Hernandez-Reif 1998).

5. *Urine samples for serotonin, cortisol and catecholamines.* Participants provided a urine sample on the first and last days of the 5-week study. The samples were frozen and subsequently sent to Duke University to be assayed for serotonin (5-HIAA), cortisol, catecholamines (norepinephrine, epinephrine), and dopamine. Based on earlier massage therapy studies, increased serotonin and dopamine (Field, Grizzle, Scafidi & Schanberg 1996) and decreased cortisol and catecholamines (Field et al 1992) were expected for the massage group by the last day of the study.

*Results*

Data analyses on the *pre/post-session measures (immediate effects)* taken on first and last days of the study revealed the following (see Table 2.14):

1. a decrease in pain intensity (on the Vitas Pain Scale) only for the massage therapy group on both the first and last days of the study
2. lower stress hormone levels (salivary cortisol) after the last session but only for the massage group.

Data analyses on the *first/last-day session measures (longer-term effects)* revealed (see Table 2.14):

1. fewer somatic symptoms and lower anxiety score (on the SCL-90-R) on the last versus the first day of the study but only for the massage group
2. a lower Global Headache Score, a greater percentage of days without headaches, and fewer days with mild head pain for the massage group (see Table 2.15). These findings suggest that the effects of massage on headache may have been limited to the reduction of mild head pain that yielded an increase in headache-free days
3. a reduction in analgesics only for the massage group
4. an increase in hours slept and a decrease in nightwakings by the last day of the study (see Table 2.15)
5. an increase in serotonin levels for the massage group over the course of the study (see Table 2.16).

**Table 2.14** Means for massage group and control group (standard deviations in parentheses) for pre/post-sessions and first/last days measures on the pain and psychological variables (Study 6)

| | Massage group ($N = 12$) | | | | Control group ($N = 14$) | | | |
|---|---|---|---|---|---|---|---|---|
| | First day | | Last day | | First day | | Last day | |
| Variables | Pre | Post | Pre | Post | Pre | Post | Pre | Post |
| *Stress* | | | | | | | | |
| Pain (Vitas)[1] | 3.4 (2.7) | 1.4 (1.3)*** | 2.2 (2.3) | 1.0 (2.1)**** | 2.3 (2.8) | 2.3 (2.8) | 1.9 (2.1) | 2.3 (1.9) |
| Saliva (cortisol) | 1.4 (0.5) | 1.1 (0.7) | 1.1 (0.5) | 0.8 (0.4)* | 0.9 (0.6) | 0.9 (0.5) | 1.5 (1.5) | 1.3 (0.6) |
| *Longer-term measures* | | | | | | | | |
| SCL-90-R[1] | | | | | | | | |
| Somatization | | 59.1  (7.2) | | 55.5  (9.2)** | | 58.5 (10.2) | | 56.2  (9.5) |
| Depression | | 53.7 (10.4) | | 50.7 (10.7) | | 59.2 (12.7) | | 55.0 (11.0) |
| Anxiety | | 56.3  (9.9) | | 49.5 (11.3)*** | | 58.5 (15.6) | | 55.0 (13.7) |
| Hostility | | 52.7  (8.2) | | 48.3  (8.9) | | 55.9  (9.7) | | 55.2 (11.8) |

[1] Lower score is optimal.
Asterisks indicate level of significance for adjacent mean: * $p < 0.05$; ** $p < 0.01$; *** $p < 0.005$; **** $p < 0.001$.

**Table 2.15** Means (standard deviations in parentheses) for Global Headache Score (GHS) and Percentage of Days Score (PDS), medication and sleep logs for massage group versus control group (Study 6)

| Variables | Massage | Control | Effect size |
|---|---|---|---|
| | First day | Last day | |
| *Headache Log* | | | |
| Global Headache Score (GHS) | 0.79 (0.5) | 0.84 (0.5) | 0.21[1] |
| *% of Days Score (PDS)* | | | |
| % No headache | 57.6 (21.9) | 44.2 (28.7) | 0.47[2] |
| % Mild | 19.9 (13.9) | 32.8 (15.9) | 0.81[3] |
| % Moderate | 16.3 (13.3) | 15.6 (14.7) | 0.04 |
| % Severe | 6.1 (6.9) | 6.6 (7.7) | −0.07 |
| *Medication log* | *First/last day* | *First/last day* | |
| Analgesics | 1.5/0.7* | 0.8/0.8 | |
| *Sleep log* | | | |
| # of hours slept | 6.0/7.5*** | 7.5/7.8 | |
| # of night wakings | 1.4/0.6* | 2.4/2.7 | |

Asterisks indicate level of significance for adjacent mean: * $p$ <0.05; ** $p$ <0.01; *** $p$ < 0.005.
[1] = small effect; [2] = moderate effect; [3] = large effect.

**Table 2.16** Means (standard deviations in parentheses) for massage group versus control group on urinary biochemical measures for first versus last day (Study 6)

| | Massage | | Control | |
|---|---|---|---|---|
| | First day | Last day | First day | Last day |
| Serotonin (5-HIAA) | 2453 (639) | 2642 (424)* | 2471 (1069) | 1887 (521) |
| Norepinephrine (ng/mg) | 37.3 (19.3) | 32.9 (19.3) | 25.7 (18.3) | 20.6 (25.6) |
| Epinephrine (ng/mg) | 8.4 (5.6) | 8.0 (5.8) | 5.0 (3.9) | 7.8 (10.8) |
| Dopamine (ng/mg) | 190 (39) | 157 (95) | 152 (85) | 136 (117) |
| Cortisol (ng/mg) | 138 (43) | 139 (43) | 119 (69) | 217 (211) |

Asterisk indicates level of significance for adjacent mean: * $p$ < 0.05.

## Discussion

The self-report and salivary cortisol data converged to suggest that massage therapy immediately reduced pain and stress. Similar effects have been observed after giving massage for other pain syndromes, including fibromyalgia (Sunshine et al 1996) and lower back pain (Hernandez-Reif, Field et al 1998). Physical and psychological stressors have been known to provoke headaches (Chen 1993), and, at least in this study, massage therapy effectively alleviated both the stress and the headaches. The most important long-term effect, the Global Headache Score, reflected more headache-free days and fewer days with mild headache pain.

Fewer nightwakings noted for the massage group by the last day of the study could have derived from fewer headaches. Massage therapy has been shown to improve sleep in at least three other studies (Field et al 1992, Field & Hernandez-Reif 1998, Sunshine et al 1996). Increased restorative or deep sleep may result in lower levels of Substance P and in turn less pain (Sunshine et al 1996). Future studies might monitor sleep more closely as well as Substance P levels.

Assays of the biochemical measures revealed an increase in serotonin levels for the massage group and a decrease for the control group. This increase in urinary serotonin levels in participants receiving massage therapy may underlie their reported reduction of mild head pain. Silberstein (1992) proposed that migraine pain is influenced by serotonin neurotransmission. The massage therapy group showing increased serotonin levels is important since many current medications prescribed for headaches increase serotonin levels (e.g., sumatriptan and selective serotonin re-uptake inhibitors such as Prozac) (Jhingran et al 1996, Visser et al 1996). Although serotonergic medications alleviate headaches (Jhingran et al 1996), side effects have been reported, including chest pain, throat tightness, and panic-like symptoms (Loi et al 1996). Increased serotonin levels in the massage therapy group may have contributed to the reduction in medication intake for this group.

While the course of massage therapy applied in this preliminary study was of short duration (i.e., 5 weeks), both significant reductions in pain and significant increases in serotonin were demonstrated. More frequent massage to the head and neck that persists over a longer time span may have a greater impact on both serotonin and severe head pain.

# POTENTIAL MODELS FOR MECHANISMS OF TOUCH AND PAIN RELIEF

## Gate theory

Pain alleviation has most frequently been attributed to the Gate Theory (Melzack & Wall 1965). This theory suggests that pain can be alleviated by pressure or cold temperature because pain fibers are shorter and less myelinated than pressure and cold temperature receptors. The pressure or cold temperature stimuli are received before the pain stimulus, the gate is closed, and thus the pain stimulus is not processed.

*Serotonin*

Another possibility is increased serotonin levels after massage therapy for both infants (Field, Grizzle, Scafidi, Abrams & Richardson 1996) and adults (Hernandez-Reif, Dieter et al 1999, Ironson et al 1996). Serotonergic drugs are noted to alleviate pain, so it would not be surprising if the body's naturally produced serotonin would reduce pain.

*Sleep deficits*

Another potential theory for pain alleviation from massage therapy relates to quiet or restorative sleep. During deep sleep, somatostatin is normally released (Sunshine et al 1996). Without this substance, pain is experienced. Substance P is released when an individual is deprived of deep sleep, and it is notable for causing pain (Sunshine et al 1996). Thus, if a person is deprived of deep sleep, they may have less somatostatin and increased Substance P, either or both causing greater pain. One of the leading theories for the pain associated with fibromyalgia syndrome, for example, is the production of Substance P due to deep sleep deprivation (Sunshine et al 1996). One of the possible reasons the subjects with fibromyalgia syndrome in the Sunshine et al (1996) study experienced less pain following the massage therapy treatment period is that they were experiencing less sleep disturbance.

REFERENCES

Achterberg J, Kenner C, Lawlis GF 1988 Severe burn injury: a comparison of relaxation, imagery, and biofeedback for pain management. Journal of Mental Imagery 12:71–88

Andrasik S, Attanasio V, Banchard EB, Burke E, Kabela E, McCarran M, Blake DD, Rosenblum EL 1984 Behavioral treatment of pediatric migraine headache. In: Andrasik F (Chair) Recent Developments in the Assessment and Treatment of Headache. Paper presented at the annual meeting of the Association for the Advancement of Behavioral Therapy, Philadelphia

Andreasen NJ, Noyes R, Hartford CE 1972 Factors influencing adjustment of burn patients during hospitalization. Psychosomatic Medicine 34:517–526

Bartels EM, Danneskiold-Samse B 1986 Histologic abnormalities in muscle from patients with certain types of fibrositis. Lancet 31:755–757

Bengtsson A, Henriksson KG, Larsson J 1986 Muscle biopsy in primary fibromyalgia: light microscopical and histochemical findings. Scandinavian Journal of Rheumatology 15:1–6

Bennett RM 1993 The origin of myopain: an integrated hypothesis of focal muscle changes and sleep disturbance in patients with fibromyalgia syndrome. The Journal of Musculoskeletal Pain 1:95–112

Bertsch TD, Nagashima WL, Dykeman E, Kennell JH 1990 Labor support by first-time fathers: direct observations. Journal of Psychosomatic Obstetric Gynecology 11:251–260

Blanchard BE, Andraik F, Neff DF, Arena JG, Ahles TA, Jurish SE, Pallmeyer TP, Sauders NL, Teders SJ, Barron KD, Rodichok LD 1982 Biofeedback and relaxation training with three kinds of headache: treatment effects and their prediction. Journal of Consulting and Clinical Psychology 50(4):562–575

Boyle G 1997 Effects of menstrual cycle moods and symptoms on academic performance: a study of senior secondary school students. British Journal of Educational Psychology 67(1):37–49

Brown J 1984 Imagery coping strategies in the treatment of migraine. Pain 18(2):157–167

Cassidy JT, Petty RE 1995 Textbook of pediatric rheumatology 3rd edn. WB Saunders, Philadelphia

Chen A 1993 Headache: contrast between childhood and adult pain. International Journal of Adolescent Medicine and Health 6(2):75–93

Cohen J 1968 Weighted kappa: nominal scale agreement with provision for scaled disagreement or partial credit. Psychological Bulletin 70:213–220

Coppen A, Kessel N 1963 Menstruation and personality. British Journal of Psychiatry 109:711

Corney R, Stanton R 1991 A survey of 658 women who report symptoms of premenstrual syndrome. Journal of Psychosomatic Research 35:471–482

Cott A, Parkinson W, Fabich M, Bedard M, Marlin R 1992 Longterm efficacy of combined relaxation: biofeedback treatments for chronic headache. Pain 51:49–56

Darling M 1991 The use of exercise as a method of aborting migraine. Headache 31:616–618

Derogatis LR, 1983 SCL-90-R, administration, scoring and procedures manual II. Clinical Psychometric Research 23:118–129

Dieter JN, Swerdlow B 1988 A replicative investigation of the reliability of the MMPI in the classification of chronic headaches. Headache 28:212–222

Engelman G 1982 Labour Among Primitive Peoples. JH Chambers, St Louis

Field T 1995 Massage therapy for infants and children. Developmental and Behavioral Pediatrics 16:105–111

Field T, Hernandez-Reif M 1998 Sleep problems decrease following massage therapy. Early Child Development and Care. In press

Field T, Morrow C, Valdeon C, Larson S, Kuhn C, Schanberg S 1992 Massage reduces anxiety in child and adolescent psychiatric patients. Journal of American Academy of Child and Adolescent Psychiatry 31:125–131

Field T, Grizzle N, Scafidi F, Abrams S, Richardson S 1996 Massage therapy for infants of depressed mothers. Infant Behavior and Development 19:107–112

Field T, Grizzle N, Scafidi F, Schanberg S 1996 Massage and relaxation therapies' effects on depressed adolescent mothers. Adolescence 31:903–911.

Field T, Ironson G, Pickens J, Nawrocki T, Fox N, Scafidi F, Burman I, Schanberg S 1996 Massage therapy reduces anxiety and enhances EEG pattern of alertness and math computations. International Journal of Neuroscience 86:197–205

Field T, Seligman S, Scafidi F, Schanberg S 1996 Alleviating posttraumatic stress in children following Hurricane Andrew. Journal of Applied Developmental Psychology 17:37–50

Field T, Hernandez-Reif M, LaGreca A, Shaw K, Schanberg S, Kuhn C 1997 Glucose levels decreased after giving massage therapy to children with diabetes mellitus. Spectrum 10:23–25

Field T, Hernandez-Reif M, Seligman S, Krasnegor J, Sunshine W, Rivas-Chacon R, Schanberg S, Kuhn C 1997 Juvenile Rheumatoid Arthritis benefits from massage therapy. Journal of Pediatric Psychology 22:607–617

Field T, Hernandez-Reif M, Taylor O, Quintino O, Burman I 1997 Labor pain is reduced by massage therapy. Journal of Psychosomatic Obstetrics and Gynecology 18:186–291

Field T, Sunshine W, Hernandez-Reif M, Quintino O, Schanberg S, Kuhn C, Burman I 1997 Chronic fatigue syndrome: massage therapy effects on depression and somatic symptoms in chronic fatigue syndrome. Journal of Chronic Fatigue Syndrome 3:43–51

Field T, Henteleff T, Hernandez-Reif M, Martinez E, Mavunda J, Kuhn C Schanberg S 1998 Children with asthma have improved pulmonary function after massage therapy. Journal of Pediatrics 132:854–858

Field T, Peck M, Burman I, Krugman S 1998 Massage therapy effects on burn patients. Journal of Burn Care & Rehabilitation, 19:241–244

Fontana AM, Badawy S 1997 Perceptual and coping processes across the menstrual cycle: an investigation in a premenstrual syndrome clinic and a community sample. Behavioral Medicine 22:152–159

Freeman EW, Rickels K, Sondheimer SJ, Wittmaack FM 1996 Sertraline versus desipramine in the treatment of premenstrual syndrome: an open label trial. Journal of Clinical Psychiatry 57:7–11

Fries J, Spitz P, Young D 1982 The dimensions of health outcomes: the health assessment questionnaire, disability and pain scales. Journal of Rheumatology 9:789

Gauthier JG, Ivers H, Carrier S 1996 Nonpharmacological approaches in the management of recurrent headache disorders and their comparison and combination with pharmacotherapy. Clinical Psychology Review 16(6):543–571

Gilboa D, Bornstein A, Seidman DS, Tsur H 1990 Burn patients' use of autohypnosis: making a painful experience bearable. Burns 16:441–444

Hammill JM, Cook TM, Rosecrance JC 1996 Effectiveness of a physical therapy regimen in the treatment of tension-type headache. Headache 36:149–153

Hart KE, Hill AL 1997 Generalized use of over-the-counter analgesics: relationship to premenstrual syndrome. Journal of Clinical Psychology 53:197–200

Hedstrom LW, Newton N 1986 Touch in labor: a comparison of cultures and eras. Birth Issues in Perinatal Care and Education 13:181–186

Hernandez-Reif M, Dieter J, Field T, Diego M, Swerdlow B 1999 Massage therapy effects on headache sufferers. International Journal of Neuroscience 96:11

Hernandez-Reif M, Field T, Krasnegor J, Theakston H, Burman I 1999 Chronic low back pain is reduced and range of motion improved with massage therapy. Journal of Bodywork & Movement Therapies. In review

Hickling EJ, Silverman DJ, Loos W 1990 A non-pharmacological treatment of vascular headache during pregnancy. Headache 30:407–410

High RV, Marcellino PA 1995 Premenstrual symptoms and the female employee. Social Behavior & Personality 23:265–271

Ironson G, Field T, Scafidi F, Kumar M, Patarca R, Price A, Goncalves A, Hashimoto M, Kumar A, Burman I, Tetenman S, Fletcher M 1996 Massage therapy is associated with enhancement of the immune system's cytotoxic capacity. International Journal of Neuroscience 84:205–217

Jensen OK, Nielsen FF, Vosmar L 1990 An open study comparing manual therapy with the use of cold packs in the treatment of post-traumatic headache. Cephalagia 10:241–250

Jhingran P, Cady RK, Rubino J, et al 1996 Improvements in health-related quality of life with sumatriptan treatment for migraine. Journal of Family Practice 42:36–42

Keenan, PA, Stern RA, Ianowsky DS, Pedersen CA 1992 Psychological aspects of premenstrual syndrome I: cognition and memory. Psychoneuroendocrinology 17:179–187

Kennell J, Klaus M, McGrath S, Robertson S, Hickley C 1991 Continuous emotional support during labor in a US Hospital. Journal of American Medical Association 265:2197–2201

Kimball KL, Drews JE, Walker S, Dimick AR 1987 Use of TENS for pain reduction in burn patients. Journal of Burn Care Rehabilitation 8:28–31

King R 1995 Cadavers, swings and brain pain or guess what's causing your headache. Massage Therapy Journal 29:92–96

Korol C, Von Baeyer C 1992 Effects of brief instruction in imagery and birth visualization in prenatal education. Journal of Mental Imagery 16:167–172

Lavigne JV, Ross CK, Berry SL, Hayford JR, Pachman LM 1992 Evaluation of a psychological treatment package for treating pain in juvenile rheumatoid arthritis. Arthritis Care and Research 5:101–110

Lindberg C, Lawlis GF 1988 The effectiveness of imagery as a childbirth preparatory technique. Journal of Mental Imagery 12:103–114

Lipton SA 1986 Prevention of classic migraine headache by digital massage of the superficial temporal arteries during visual aura. Annals of Neurology 19:515–516

Littman D, Parmelee A 1978 Medical correlates of infant development. Pediatrics 61:470–482

Lockett DM, Campbell JF 1990 The effects of aerobic exercises on migraine. Headache 30:407–410

Loi V, Lai M, Pisano MR, Del Zompo M 1996 Sumatriptan and panic-like symptoms. American Journal of Psychology 153(11):1505

Lovell, Walco 1989 Pain associated with juvenile rheumatoid arthritis. Pediatric Clinics of North America 36:4

Marcus DA 1993 Serotonin and its role in headache pathogenesis and treatment. Clinical Journal of Pain 9(3):159–167

McCain GA 1989 Non-medicinal treatments in primary fibromyalgia. Rheumatic Disease Clinics of North America 15:73–90

McGrady A, Wauquier A, McNeil A, Gerard G 1994 Effect of biofeedback-assisted relaxation on migraine headache and changes in cerebral blood flow velocity in the middle cerebral artery. Headache 34:424–428

McNair DM, Lorr M 1964 An analysis of mood in neurotics. Journal of Abnormal Social Psychology 69:620–627

McNair DM, Lorr M, Droppleman LF 1971 POMS – profile of mood states. Educational and Industrial Testing Service, San Diego

Melzack R 1987 The short-form McGill Pain Questionnaire. Pain 30:191–197

Melzack R, Wall PD 1965 Pain mechanisms: a new theory. Science 150:971–978

Metcalf MG 1995 The premenstrual syndrome: a reappraisal of the concept and the evidence: comment. Psychological Medicine 25:657

Meyer JS 1993 Current concepts of headache and its treatment in the People's Republic of China. Headache Quarterly 4:163–168

Moos RH 1968 The development of a menstrual distress questionnaire. Psychosomatic Medicine 30:853–867

Morse C, Dennerstein L, Farrell E, Varnavides K 1991 A comparison of hormone therapy, coping skills training, and relaxation for the relief of premenstrual syndrome. Journal of Behavioral Medicine 14:469–489

Mueller S, Sahs AL 1976 Brain stem dysfunction related to cervical manipulation. Neurology 26:547

Nagashima L, Berschi T, Dykeman S, McGrath S, Delay T, Kennell J 1987 Fathers during labor: do we expect too much? Pediatric Research 21:

O'Neill A 1994 Danger and safety in medicines. Social Science and Medicine 38(4) 497–507

Patterson DR 1992 Practical applications of psychological techniques in controlling burn pain. Journal of Burn Care Rehabilitation 13:13–17

Pearlstein T, Rivera-Tovar A, Frank E et al 1992 Nonmedical management of late luteal phase dysphoric disorder: a preliminary report. Journal of Psychotherapy Practice and Research 1:49–55

Platania-Solazzo A, Field T, Blank J, Seligman F, Kuhn C, Schanberg S, Saab P 1992 Relaxation therapy reduces anxiety in child/adolescent psychiatry patients. Acta Paedopsychiatrica 55:115–120

Pugatch D, Haskell D, McNair DM 1969 Predictors and patterns of change associated with the course of time-limited psychotherapy. Mimeo Report

Puustjarvi K, Aoraksinen O, Pontinen PJ 1990 The effects of massage in patients with chronic tension headache. Acupuncture Electrotherapy Research 15:159–162

Radloff L 1977 The CES-D scale: a self-report depression scale for research in the general population. Applied Psychological Measures 1:385–401

Raft D, Smith M, Warren LD 1986 Selection of imagery in the relief of chronic and acute clinical pain. Journal of Psychosomatic Research 30:481–488

Rausch JL, Parry BL 1993 Treatment of premenstrual mood symptoms. Psychiatric Clinics of North America 16:829–839

Read D 1972 Childbirth without fear: the principles and practices of natural childbirth. New York Press, New York

Rivera-Tovar A, Pilknois P, Frank E 1992 Symptom patterns in late luteal-phase dysphoric disorder. Journal of Psychopathic & Behavioral Assessment 14:189–199

Royeen CB 1987 Test-retest reliability of a touch scale for tactile defensiveness. Occupational and Physical Therapy in Pediatrics 7:45–52

Rubinow D, Roy-Byrne P 1984 Premenstrual syndromes: overview from a methodological perspective. American Journal of Psychiatry 141:163–172

Russell IJ, Orr MD, Vipraio GA, Alboukrek D, Michalek JE, MacKillip F, Lopez YM, Littman BH 1993 Cerebrospinal fluid substance P is elevated in fibromyalgia syndrome. Arthritis and Rheumatism 36:223

Saper JR, Silberstein SD, Gordon CD, Hamel RL, 1995 Handbook of headache management: a practical guide to diagnosis and treatment of head, neck and facial pain. Williams & Wilkins, Baltimore, pp 93–95

Silberstein SD 1992 Advances in understanding the pathophysiology of headache. Neurology 42:6–10

Simms RW 1994 Muscle studies in fibromyalgia syndrome. Journal of Musculoskeletal Pain 2:117–123

Sosa, R, Kennell, J, Klaus, M, Urrutia, J 1980 The effect of a supportive companion on perinatal problems, length of labor, and mother infant interaction. New England Journal of Medicine 303:597–600

Spielberger CD 1972 Anxiety as an emotional state. In: Spielberger CD (ed) Anxiety: current trends in theory and research. Academic Press, New York

Spielberger CD Gorsuch RL, Lushene RE 1970 The State Trait Anxiety Inventory. Consulting Psychologists Press, Palo Alto, CA

Steiner M 1996 Premenstrual dysphoric disorder: an update. General Hospital Psychiatry 18(4):244–250

Stolte KM 1976 An exploratory study of patient perceptions of the touch they receive during labor. Unpublished dissertation

Stout A, Steege J 1985 Psychological assessment of women seeking treatment for premenstrual syndrome. Journal of Psychosomatic Research 29:621–629

Sundblad, C, Modigh, K, Andersch, B, et al 1992 Clomipramine effectively reduces premenstrual syndrome. British Medical Journal 305:346–347

Sunshine W, Field T, Schanberg S, Quintino O, Kilmer T, Fierro K, Burman I, Hashimoto M, McBride C, Henteleff T 1996 Massage therapy and transcutaneous electrical stimulation effects on fibromyalgia. Journal of Clinical Rheumatology 2:18–22

Swerdlow B, Dieter JN 1989 The vascular "cold patch" is not a prognostic index for headache. Headache 29:562–568

Takeshima T, Shimomura T, Takahashi K 1987 Platelet activation in muscle contraction headache and migraine. Cephalalgia 7(4):239–243

ter Kuile M, Spinhoven P, Linsser AC, Van Houwelingen HC 1995 Cognitive coping and appraisal processes in the treatment of chronic headaches. Pain 64:257–264

Vaeroy H, Helle R, Forre O, Kass E, Terenius, L 1988 Elevated CSF levels of substance P and high incidence of Raynoud's phenomenon in patients with fibromyalgia: new features for diagnosis. Pain 32:21–26

Van Der Meer A 1990 Relief from chronic headaches. Dell Publishing, New York

Varni JW, Bernstein BH 1991 Evaluation and management of pain in children with rheumatic diseases. Rheumatic Disease Clinics of North America 17:4

Varni JW, Jay SM 1984 Biobehavioral factors in juvenile rheumatoid arthritis: implications for research and practice. Clinical Psychology Review 4:543

Varni JW, Thompson KL, Hanson V 1987 The Varni/Thompson Pediatric Pain Questionnaire, I: chronic musculoskeletal pain in juvenile rheumatoid arthritis. Pain 28:27–38

Vernon HT 1995 The effectiveness of chiropractic manipulation in the treatment of headache: an exploration in the literature. Journal of Manipulative Physiology Therapy 18(9):611–617

Visser W, Hester V, Rolf HM, Jaspers NM, Ferrar MD 1996 Sumatriptan in clinical practice: a 2-year review of 453 migraine patients. Neurology 47(1):46–51

Walco GA, Varni JW, Ilowite NT 1992 Cognitive behavioral pain management in children with juvenile rheumatoid arthritis. Pediatrics 89:1075–1079

Wall PD, Melzack R 1984 Textbook of pain. Churchill Livingstone, New York

Wauquier A, McGrady A, Aloe L, Klausner T, Collins B 1995 Changes in cerebral blood flow velocity associated with biofeedback-assisted relaxation treatment of migraine headaches are specific for the middle cerebral artery. Headache 35:358–362

Wideman MV, Singer JE 1984 The role of psychological mechanisms in preparation for childbirth. American Psychologist 39:1357–1371

Wood SH, Mortola JF, Yuen-Fai C et al 1992 Treatment of premenstrual syndrome with fluoxetine: a double-blind, placebo-controlled, crossover study. Obstetric Gynecology 80:339–344

Yunus MB, Masi AT 1985 Juvenile primary fibromyalgia syndrome: A clinical study of thirty-three patients and matched normal controls. Arthritis and Rheumatism 28:138–145

# Enhancing attentiveness

Sleep deprivation, lower vagal activity, or some other mediating mechanism might also contribute to attentional problems such as autism and attention deficit disorder, and massage therapy appears to help these as well. Our studies combined with studies by Dember and colleagues (Warm, Dember & Parasuraman 1991) on enhancing attentiveness by aroma stimulation suggest that multiple forms of stimulation (therapies) are effective. Again, the accumulating empirical data highlight the need for mechanism studies.

Attention deficits like autism and attention deficit disorder in children are very disruptive of classroom behavior and learning. Very little is known about the etiology of these disorders, but some behavioral management techniques and some arousal-reducing therapies like massage seem to have positive effects.

## ATTENTION DEFICITS IN AUTISM

### Study 1: Children with autism – attentiveness and responsivity improved after touch therapy

Autism affects two to five of 10 000 children. Although once considered primarily psychiatric in nature, autism is now generally thought to be an organic defect in brain development. Characterized

by a failure to develop language or other forms of social communication, symptoms of autism include:

1. withdrawal from or failure to develop normal relationships
   with people
2. abnormal responses to one or more types of sensory stimuli
   (usually sound)
3. atypical movement, including immobility and hyperkinesis
4. limited attention span and excessive off-task behavior
5. touch aversion.

A variety of therapies have been tried with children with autism,
including structured activities, behavior modification, sensori-
motor and sensory integrative approaches. Touch therapy may
also be beneficial for children with autism. Previous studies, for
example, have shown that touch therapy alleviated anxiety and
decreased cortisol levels and depression in child psychiatric
patients (Field et al 1992). In another study, vagal activity increased
during touch therapy (Field 1990). Since increased vagal activity
has been associated with increased attention span (Porges 1991),
touch therapy may reduce the off-task behavior noted in autistic
children. This study investigated the effects of touch therapy on
three problems commonly associated with autism: inattentiveness
(off-task behavior), touch aversion, and withdrawal.

## Method

**Sample** The subjects were 22 preschool children (12 boys) with
autism (diagnosed by two independent clinicians using DSM-
III-R criteria) who had attended a special preschool half days for
2 years. The program offered model preschool activities including
story time, free play, arts and crafts, and gross motor play on the
playground. The children averaged 4.5 years of age and were
from middle socioeconomic status families. They were randomly
assigned to a touch therapy or a touch control group based on a
stratification procedure to ensure equivalence between groups.
The children also continued with their normal school curriculum
during this study.

**Procedure**

*Touch therapy.* The children assigned to this group received
touch therapy from a volunteer student for 15 minutes per day,
2 days per week for a period of 4 weeks (eight therapy sessions).
The children were fully clothed (except for the removal of shoes
and socks), and their body was rubbed using moderate pressure
and smooth stroking movements on each of the following areas:

head/neck, arms/hands, torso, and legs/feet. The volunteer student stroked five regions of the child's body in the following sequence:

1. *face*:
   (a) six strokes along both sides of the face using the flats of the fingers and proceeding from the temples to the jawbone
   (b) six strokes with the flats of the fingers across the forehead, proceeding from the center of the forehead to the temples
   (c) one series of circular strokes over the temples proceeding downward to the hinge of the jaw using fingertips
   (d) two strokes placing the flats of the fingers and the palms of the hand over the nose, cheeks, jaw, and chin simultaneously, proceeding from the bridge of the nose to the jawline

2. *chest*:
   (a) six strokes on both sides of the chest with the flats of the fingers, going from midline outward
   (b) six cross strokes from center of chest and going over the shoulders
   (c) two strokes on sides of the chest toward the shoulders

3. *stomach*:
   (a) six hand-over-hand strokes in a paddlewheel fashion, avoiding the ribs and the tip of the rib cage
   (b) one series of circular motions with fingertips in a clockwise direction starting at the appendix and proceeding along the large intestine

4. *legs*:
   (a) six strokes with the flats of the fingertips on the front of the leg beginning at the ankle and proceeding to the hip; continue strokes over outside of the leg back to the ankle
   (b) two strokes with the flats of the fingers from the hip to the foot

5. *foot*:
   (a) using the fingers for support, firm circles with the thumbs on the bottom of the foot using a continuous movement lasting approximately 15 seconds
   (b) criss-crossing the thumbs along the bottom of the foot in a 10-second continuous movement
   (c) squeezing each toe between the index finger and thumb and pulling lightly

6. *arms*:
   (a) holding the child's wrist in one hand and with the other hand stroking the arm from the wrist to the shoulder, repeating six times

(b) holding the child's arm with palm down and using thumbs to make circular strokes on the top of the hand for approximately 10 seconds

(c) repeating above motion for palm of the hand, holding the child's arm with the palm of the hand facing up

(d) squeezing each finger between the index finger and the thumb and pulling.

The child was placed in a prone position for the second phase, and the *back* massaged in the following sequence:

(a) six downward strokes along the back using the flats of the fingers

(b) continuous hand-over-hand movements down the back, proceeding to the waist

(c) using palms of hands to spread out the back from spine to sides; working up and down the back twice

(d) circular motions from the neck to the tailbone along one side of the spine; crossing over the spine and going up the other side of the back toward the neck; making two complete cycles

(e) rubbing and kneading shoulder muscles for 10 seconds

(f) rubbing the neck for 10 seconds using the flats of the fingers

(h) two strokes along the length of the back using the fingertips and proceeding from the neck to the tailbone.

*Touch control group.* For the touch control group a volunteer student sat with the child on her lap with her arms around the child and engaged the child in a game selecting different color/form/shape toys. The control group sessions were also held for 15 minutes per day 2 days per week for 4 weeks.

**Assessments** The children's scores on developmental assessments were first examined to ensure that the two groups were equivalent. The average scores were as follows:

1. The preschool IQ (Preschool Performance Scale) averaged 91.

2. The speech and language evaluation scores (Sequenced Inventory of Communication Development) averaged 20 months for receptive and 16 months for expressive language.

3. The Vineland Adaptive Behavior Scale composite scores averaged 64.

The therapy and control group children did not differ on these baseline measures.

To assess the effects of the touch therapy, the children from both groups were assessed on the first day and the last day of the study by being

1. observed in their classrooms for touch aversion, off-task behavior, orienting to irrelevant sounds, and stereotypic behaviors
2. assessed by their teachers on the Autism Behavior Checklist (Krug, Arick, & Almond 1979) based on the teachers' observations of the children
3. given the Early Social Communication Scales (ESCS) (Seibert, Hogan, & Mundy 1982) by psychology graduate students.

The classroom observations were conducted for 30 minutes per child on the first and last days of the study using 10-second time sample unit coding sheets. The psychology graduate student observers were blind to the children's group assignment. The behaviors observed included touch aversion, off-task behavior, orienting to irrelevant sounds, and stereotypic behaviors.

For the ESCS, the child and a tester sat facing each other at a small table. A set of toys – a hat, a comb, a picture book, a ball, a car, and three small wind-up mechanical toys – were in view, but out of reach of the child. Throughout the course of the ESCS, the tester presented each of the toys. This procedure was videotaped to record the tester and child. The period of interaction with each child was approximately 20 minutes. The ESCS scale was used because one of its authors had previously reported joint attention disturbances in children with autism (Mundy, Sigman, & Kasari 1994).

## Results

Analyses of the classroom observation data revealed the following (see Table 3.1).

1. Touch aversion decreased in both the touch therapy and the touch control group.

2. Off-task behavior decreased in both groups but significantly more for the massage group.

3. Orienting to irrelevant sounds decreased for both groups, but significantly more in the touch therapy group.

4. Stereotypic behaviors decreased in both groups but significantly more in the touch therapy group.

Data analyses of the Autism Behavior Checklist revealed that only the children in the touch therapy group changed. These changes included significant decreases (decreases being optimal) on (1) the sensory scale, (2) the relating scale, and (3) the total scale score. Finally, data analyses revealed significant changes on the Early Social Communication Scales, but again only for the touch therapy group, including improvements in (1) joint attention, (2) behavior regulation, (3) social behavior, and (4) initiating behavior.

## Discussion

That both groups improved on some behaviors, notably touch aversion and off-task behavior, is probably not surprising given that both interventions involved additional one-on-one attention and physical contact from an adult. Surprisingly, although touch aversion has been anecdotally reported for children with autism, the children did not seem aversive to the touch therapy or the lap sitting even initially. This may have related to both forms of physical contact being more predictable than social touch in general. The more active physical contact and relaxation involved in the touch therapy may have contributed to the many ways in which the touch therapy children were advantaged, including showing

**Table 3.1** Mean change scores for touch therapy and touch control groups (Study 1)

| | Groups | | |
| --- | --- | --- | --- |
| Variables | Touch therapy | Touch control | Optimal direction |
| *Classroom observations* | | | |
| Touch aversion | $-2.6_a$* | $-3.0_a$* | neg. |
| Off-task behavior | $-12.8_a$* | $-12.3_a$* | neg. |
| Orienting to irrelevant sounds | $-2.1_a$* | $-0.7_b$* | neg. |
| Stereotypical behaviors | $-8.2_a$* | $-0.3_b$* | neg. |
| *Autism behavior checklist* | | | |
| Sensory | $-2.4_a$* | $-0.4_b$ | neg. |
| Relating | $-3.2_a$* | $1.3_b$ | neg. |
| Object use | $-2.3_a$ | $-2.4_a$ | neg. |
| Language | $-1.1_a$ | $-0.4_a$ | neg. |
| Social skills | $-2.4_a$ | $-1.7_a$ | neg. |
| Total | $-10.6_a$ | $-5.0_b$ | neg. |
| *Early social communication scales* | | | |
| Joint attention | $2.3_a$* | $-2.5_b$ | pos. |
| Behavior regulation | $6.3_a$* | $-0.5_b$ | pos. |
| Social | $5.0_a$* | $1.8_b$ | pos. |
| Initiating | $2.3_a$* | $-1.3_b$ | pos. |

* Significant changes (@ $p < 0.05$) from beginning to end of therapy. When one group changes significantly more than the other (@ $p < 0.05$) the values have different subscripts.

fewer autistic behaviors (orienting to sounds and stereotypic behaviors) and improvement on social relating as measured on the Autism Behavior Checklist and the Early Social Communication Scales.

The increased attentiveness noted during the classroom behavior observations and on the Early Social Communication Scales could be related to enhanced vagal activity that occurs during touch therapy (Field 1990). Another related finding is that EEG patterns change in the direction of heightened alertness, and math performance improves in adults following touch therapy (Field, Ironson et al 1996). The use of these measures (vagal tone and EEG) in future studies might help explain the relationship between touch therapy and the important changes in touch aversion, off-task behavior, and social withdrawal noted in these preschool children with autism.

## ATTENTION DEFICIT HYPERACTIVITY DISORDER

Children with Attention Deficit Hyperactivity Disorder (ADHD) experience problems staying on task in the classroom. In a recent study, ADHD adolescents were provided massage therapy or relaxation therapy for 10 consecutive school days (Field, Quintino et al 1998). The massage therapy group, compared with the relaxation therapy group, showed less fidgeting behavior following the sessions. In addition, after the 2-week period, their teachers (who were blind to the group assignments) reported that the children spent more time on task and were less hyperactive in the classroom.

### Study 2: ADHD adolescents benefit from massage therapy

ADHD is a condition affecting as many as 3–6% of all youth, and is characterized by developmentally inappropriate degrees of inattention, impulsiveness, and hyperactivity. Overactivity is typically the most prominent feature (DSM-III-R, American Psychiatric Association 1987, Anderson et al 1987).

Treatment is made more difficult by the comorbidity of ADHD with other disorders, such as conduct disorder, anxiety, learning disability, and depression (Biederman, Newcorn & Spirch 1991). Treatment usually includes drug therapy and training parents and teachers in behavior modification techniques. Drug therapy features psychostimulants, such as methylphenidate or d-amphetamine, which alter the concentration and physiology of the catecholamine dopamine (Barkley 1989, Evans, Gualtieri &

Hicks 1986). This stimulates the frontal and striatal regions of the brain, which are associated with attention, arousal and inhibition and help regulate these processes (Evans et al 1986). Although drug therapy improves ADHD symptoms in over 75% of the cases, it is not a curative measure, its effects lasting only as long as medication is taken. Another drawback of drug therapy is the occasional side effects such as appetite loss and insomnia (Barkley et al 1989).

Behavior modification by parents and teachers involves techniques such as adjusting the time, amplitude, and frequency of consequences for the child's actions, rearranging home and classroom settings to facilitate attention, breaking down tasks into smaller subtasks that can be completed within the child's attention span, and setting up schedules to aid in the child's organizational problems (DSM-III-R, American Psychiatric Association 1987). Behavior modification is a way to adjust the surrounding to facilitate the ADHD child's performance. However, as with drug therapies, behavior modification is only effective during the time that the therapy is administered.

Alternative forms of therapy, namely massage therapy and relaxation therapy, were investigated in the present study because they have been effective with other children and adolescents with attention problems. Relaxation therapy (Platania-Solazzo et al 1992) and massage therapy (Field et al 1992), for example, led to reduced anxiety and activity levels in child and adolescent psychiatric patients. In addition, following massage, they had more organized sleep and lower stress hormone (cortisol and norepinephrine) levels. Massage therapy was also noted to decrease off-task behavior in children with autism, as in the study just presented (Field, Lasko et al 1996). In a similar way, massage therapy was expected to lower the level of activity in adolescents with ADHD.

## Method

**Sample** Subjects were 28 adolescents (mean age = 14.6) recruited from self-contained classrooms for emotionally disturbed adolescents. All subjects were male, most were middle socioeconomic status (90%), and they were distributed 29% non-White Hispanic and 71% White. All subjects were diagnosed with ADHD according to the DSM-III-R criteria. Subjects were randomly assigned to massage therapy or relaxation therapy based on a stratification procedure to ensure equivalence between groups on age, sex, and socioeconomic status. The groups did not differ on these background variables.

## Procedure

*Massage therapy.* The massage therapy subjects received a 15-minute massage after school for 10 consecutive school days. The massage consisted of moderate pressure and smooth strokes for 5 minutes in each of three regions: up and down the neck, from the neck across the shoulders and back to the neck, and from the neck to the waist and back to the neck along the vertebral column. The 15-minute sequence was composed of 30 back and forth strokes per region, at 10 seconds each.

*Relaxation therapy.* The relaxation therapy subjects also participated in 15-minute sessions after school for 10 consecutive days. During their progressive muscle relaxation sessions a therapist asked the adolescents to tense and relax the same body parts that were massaged in the massage therapy group.

## Assessments

*Pre/post-therapy session measures.* These included the *Happy Face Scale* completed by the adolescent and an assessment of *Fidgeting* based on a behavioral observation made by an observer who was blind to the child's group assignment. The Happy Face scale (Appendix 3A) is a series of four drawings ranging from unhappy to happy faces, used as a 'barometer' to depict the adolescents' feelings before and after the sessions. Fidgeting was rated on a 3-point scale as one of the most characteristic problems of this group of adolescents.

*First-day/last-day assessments.* Included self-report measures of *depression* and *empathy* since depression and antisocial behavior are often comorbid with ADHD (Biederman et al 1991). The *Center for Epidemiology Studies–Depression Scale* (CES–D) (Radloff 1977) was used for the adolescents' self-report on depression. The *Empathy Scale* (Bryant 1982) was adapted by our group from the Mehrabian & Epstein (1972) adult empathy scale. It requires the children to answer whether they agree or disagree with each of 22 statements designed to tap empathy, as defined by ability to take another person's perspective. It contains questions such as 'It's hard for me to see why someone else gets upset'.

*Teachers' assessments.* These included observed *time on task* in the classroom and the *Conners Scale* (Conners 1985) on the first and last days of the study. This is a 10-item scale that identifies behavior problems in children 3 to 17 years old.

## Results

Data analyses suggested the following *pre/post-therapy changes* (see Table 3.2).

1. The massage therapy group selected happier faces after than before the sessions on both the first and last days of the study.

2. The massage therapy group was observed to show less fidgeting after than before the sessions.

Data analyses yielded the following *first-day/last-day changes*.

1. The massage therapy adolescents averaged more time on task in the classroom as observed by their teachers.
2. The massage therapy group received significantly better scores on the Conners Scale.
3. No changes were noted on the depression or empathy scales.

## Discussion

While drug therapy and behavior modification techniques are commonly employed to treat ADHD, their limited effects led to this investigation of two alternative therapies: relaxation and massage therapy. The positive effects of massage therapy in this study were perhaps not surprising inasmuch as that massage has helped reduce depression and anxiety levels as well as stress hormones in child and adolescent psychiatry patients (Field et al 1992) and has enhanced on-task behavior in children with autism (Field et al 1996). Although the ADHD comorbid problems of depression and lack of empathy were not altered in this study, the adolescents reported feeling better (happier) after their massage

**Table 3.2** Means for pre/post massage and relaxation sessions[1] measures for first and last days (Study 2)

| Measure | First day | | Last day | |
| --- | --- | --- | --- | --- |
| | Pre | Post | Pre | Post |
| Happy Face | 2.8$_a$ | 3.9$_b$ | 2.9$_a$ | 3.5$_b$ |
| | 3.2 | 3.3 | 3.1 | 3.2 |
| Fidgeting | 2.7$_a$ | 3.0$_b$ | 2.5$_a$ | 3.0$_b$ |
| | 2.6 | 2.3 | 2.2 | 2.6 |
| | **First day** | | **Last day** | |
| CESD[2] | 10.2 | | 13.8 | |
| | 15.6 | | 14.7 | |
| Empathy[2] | 12.4 | | 11.2 | |
| | 11.3 | | 12.4 | |
| % time on task | 43.4$_a$ | | 76.7$_b$ | |
| | 40.5 | | 51.2 | |
| Conners Scale[2] | 28.0$_a$ | | 11.3$_b$ | |
| | 19.6 | | 28.5 | |

[1] Data for the relaxation sessions are in the lower row of each pair of rows.
[2] Lower score is optimal.
Different subscripts denote significant differences between adjacent columns.

therapy sessions, and they were observed to fidget less. Longer-term effects were reported by their teachers, including more time on task in the classroom and lower 'hyperactivity' scores on the teacher's Conners Scale.

Since hyperactivity, not depression, is the salient problem in ADHD, it is interesting that hyperactivity was uniquely reduced in this study. Although the underlying mechanism for the relationship between massage therapy and lesser activity is not known, increased serotonin levels noted in other massage studies (Field, Ironson et al 1996, Ironson et al 1996) might help modulate elevated dopamine levels noted in ADHD youth (Rogeness, Javors & Pliszka 1992) and lower the activity associated with elevated dopamine. Future studies might assay dopamine levels as well as its known regulators, norepinephrine and serotonin.

Although relaxation therapy has been effective with depressed adolescents (Platania-Solazzo et al 1992), no changes were noted following relaxation therapy in the present study. The lack of effects may relate to the adolescents 'not enjoying the relaxation therapy', as several of them reported during the course of the study. This more active form of therapy was labeled 'hard work' by those who complained.

Although the underlying mechanism for the massage therapy effects on ADHD is not known, that form of therapy could become an important tool in the management of ADHD, in conjunction with currently used therapies. It may, for example, potentiate the positive effects of methylphenidate and other drugs and/or complement the effects of behavior modification. In cases where present therapies are not effective or are accompanied by undesirable side effects, massage therapy could be an effective substitute treatment for children diagnosed with ADHD.

## Study 3: ADHD benefits from Tai Chi

As already discussed in Study 2, ADHD is characterized by cognitive and behavioral deficits including inattention, impulsivity, and hyperactivity (DSM-III-R, American Psychiatric Association 1987). Although short-term improvements have been reported in academic and social functioning with drug therapy such as methylphenidate or Ritalin (Schachar & Tannock 1983, Swanson et al 1995), side effects such as motor tics, insomnia, headaches, and social withdrawal make this treatment controversial (Handen et al 1991, Parraga & Cochran 1992).

Nonpharmacological treatments include counseling, parent/family training in behavior modification techniques, and relaxation and massage therapy. Counseling treatments have received little empirical attention, and reports are mostly anecdotal (Schwiebert, Sealander & Tollerud 1995). Behavior modification techniques have attempted to facilitate the child's performance and attention by including scheduling changes, rearranging home and classroom settings, and training teachers, parents, and siblings in differential reinforcement techniques (Blakemore, Shindler & Conte 1993). Although some studies have shown that behavioral modification is effective (Damico & Armstrong 1996), one study showed that ADHD adolescents had a weak behavioral inhibition system (Iaboni, Douglas & Ditto 1997), which made them poor candidates for behavioral programs. Although relaxation therapy has alleviated depression in adolescents (Platania-Solazzo et al 1992), it had limited effects in treating adolescents with ADHD in the study just presented (Field, Quintino et al 1998), perhaps because of the demands that relaxation therapy places on concentration. In contrast, as noted in Study 2, massage therapy, in the same study that increased the time adolescents spent on task, reduced their fidgeting, improved their mood, and lowered their hyperactivity (Field et al 1998).

Tai Chi has been effective with adults by reducing stress and stress hormones (Jin 1992), anger and confusion, and improving mood (Brown et al 1995, Wolf et al 1996). In the present study, Tai Chi was expected to reduce anxiety, depressed mood, hyperactivity, and conduct problems in adolescents with ADHD.

## Method

**Sample** Thirteen adolescents (11 males) with a mean age of 14.5 years (range = 13–16) and a DSM-III-R diagnosis of ADHD were recruited from a remedial school for adolescents with developmental problems. The adolescents came from middle class families (mean = 2.2 on Hollingshead Two Index Factor) and were ethnically distributed 70% Caucasian, 15% Hispanic, and 15% African American.

**Procedure**

*Tai Chi.* The adolescents engaged in Tai Chi postures for 30-minute sessions twice a week for 5 weeks. Each midafternoon session began with slow raising and lowering of the arms in synchrony with breathing exercises for 5 minutes. The adolescents were then taught to perform slow turning and twisting movements of the arms and legs, shifting body weight from one leg to the other, rotating from side to side, and changing directions in a sequence of Tai Chi forms.

A baseline phase of 1 week without Tai Chi was followed by a 5-week Tai Chi phase and a 2-week follow-up phase without Tai Chi. At the end of each phase, the teachers, who were not aware of which adolescents were participating in Tai Chi at what time, completed the Conners Teacher Rating Scale.

*Conners Teacher Rating Scale – Revised* (CTRS–R) (Goyette, Conners & Ulrich 1978). This 28-item teacher rating scale yields a total hyperactivity score in addition to the subcategories of anxiety, asocial behavior, conduct, daydreaming, emotion and hyperactivity.

## Results

Data analyses suggested the following baseline to Tai Chi therapy changes (see Table 3.3):

1. less anxiety
2. improved conduct
3. less daydreaming
4. less inappropriate emotions
5. less hyperactivity during Tai Chi than before Tai Chi

These improved scores persisted over the 2-week follow-up (no Tai Chi) period.

## Discussion

The results of this study and our earlier massage therapy study (Field, Quintino et al 1998) suggest that at least two nondrug therapies are effective for adolescents with ADHD. The positive effects of Tai Chi on the adolescents with ADHD parallel the

**Table 3.3**    Means (and standard deviations in parentheses) on Conners Teacher Rating Scale for baseline, Tai Chi and 2-week follow-up period (Study 3)

| Variables | Baseline first day | Tai Chi last day | No Tai Chi 2 weeks later | F | p |
|---|---|---|---|---|---|
| Conners |  |  |  |  |  |
| Anxiety | $56.7(11.3)_a$ | $43.5\ (9.6)_b$*** | $44.5\ (6.3)_b$*** | 11.94 | 0.000 |
| Asocial | $52.3(15.2)_a$ | $46.5\ (9.7)_a$ | $48.7(10.9)_a$ | 1.42 | 0.262 |
| Conduct | $56.2\ (8.0)_a$ | $49.0(11.8)_b$* | $50.5(11.9)_b$* | 5.18 | 0.013 |
| Daydream | $61.0\ (6.4)_a$ | $48.4(11.6)_b$*** | $50.5\ (7.0)_b$*** | 13.75 | 0.000 |
| Emotion | $60.4\ (8.9)_a$ | $50.2(13.5)_b$** | $52.0(12.3)_b$** | 9.04 | 0.001 |
| Hyperactive | $60.1\ (7.9)_a$ | $45.8(10.1)_b$**** | $51.7\ (8.2)_b$**** | 23.25 | 0.000 |
| Total | $81.5(11.6)_a$ | $58.6(17.8)_b$**** | $66.2(13.9)_b$**** | 19.49 | 0.000 |

Lower score is optimal.
Different letter subscript indicates significantly different means. Asterisks indicate level of significant difference between first and last days and between first day and 2 weeks later based on Bonferroni *t*-test: * $p < 0.05$; ** $p < 0.01$; *** $p < 0.005$; **** $p < 0.001$.

positive effects for adults, including reduced mental and emotional stress (Jin 1992) and improved mood (Jin 1989). Although stress hormone levels were not assayed in this study, the adolescents were perceived by their teachers as being less anxious, emotional, and hyperactive following Tai Chi. The adult literature has reported reduced stress hormones (cortisol) with Tai Chi (Jin 1992).

Tai Chi research on adults has identified changes in cardiovascular, respiratory, electroencephalographic, and biochemical levels (e.g., lower cortisol stress hormone levels) (Brown et al 1989, Jin 1989). Reduced sympathetic activity, or enhanced parasympathetic activity, has been considered a potential underlying mechanism (Hsu, Wang & Kappagoda 1985). This mechanism might also account for the marked behavioral changes observed in the adolescents in this study and in our earlier ADHD massage study (Field et al 1998). The lower stress hormone (cortisol) observed following at least the massage therapy in our other studies (Field, Seligman et al 1996, Ironson et al 1996) is consistent with a mechanism of enhanced parasympathetic activity.

Future studies might compare Tai Chi and massage therapy effects on the reduction of stress hormones (e.g., salivary cortisol or urinary catecholamines) in ADHD adolescents. The comorbidity of ADHD with other psychiatric disorders, such as depression and anxiety, and the potential side effects of a multidrug therapy, make Tai Chi and massage therapy attractive alternative treatments. In addition to little or no side effects, especially appealing are the documented effects of Tai Chi and massage therapy on reducing anxiety and hyperactivity, the major and most difficult symptoms in ADHD children.

## ALERTNESS

### Study 4: Massage therapy reduces anxiety and enhances EEG pattern of alertness and math computation performance

Despite the increasing popularity of stress-management programs (Ivancevitch et al 1990), very little evaluation research has been done. Most evaluations are based on 'professional opinions' and survey studies rather than empirical studies. A recent study on stress in HIV-positive men suggested that those who were most stressed gained most from a massage therapy intervention (Ironson et al 1996). Long-term (1 month) effects indicated immunological benefits including increased natural killer cell number and natural killer cell cytotoxicity. Massage therapy has also been noted to decrease anxiety and depression as well as cortisol and norepinephrine levels and improve sleep patterns in adolescents with psychiatric problems (Field et al 1992). Thus, massage is noted to decrease anxiety and depression based on self-report, negative behavior based on observations, salivary cortisol and urinary norepinephrine levels, and to enhance immune function.

In the above studies, subjects anecdotally reported enhanced alertness instead of the expected soporific effect following massage. The purpose of the present study was to investigate the effects of massage on alertness as measured by EEG and by speed and accuracy of performance on math computations. The only massage study in the literature that recorded EEG showed that *facial massage* was accompanied by decreased alpha and beta, a pattern that is inconsistent with drowsiness (Jodo et al 1988). The EEG alpha was expected to similarly decrease during the chair massage in this study, and the behavioral measure of alertness, namely math computation performance, was expected to improve follow-ing massages. In addition, anxiety, depression, and cortisol levels were expected to decrease as they did in the Field et al (1992) study on disturbed adolescents and the Ironson et al (1996) study on HIV-positive men.

## Method

**Sample**  The subjects were 50 medical faculty and staff members (80% females, mean age = 26). The subjects were well-educated (62% college graduate, 12% graduate school, 27% graduate degree). Income was less than $20 000 for 58%, $20–30 000 for 35%, and greater than $30 000 for 8%. Forty-six percent of the sample exer-cised regularly, with moderate numbers exercising once per week (31%), to several times per week (27%), to daily (15%). Fifty percent of the sample had tried relaxation techniques, and 62% had rarely received a massage prior to the study (62% rarely, 31% occasionally, and 8% weekly). The subjects were recruited using advertising fliers at the medical school. They were randomly assigned to the massage and the relaxation control groups. Chi square analyses comparing the two groups on sex, education, income, and lifestyle questions (i.e., exercise and previous use of massage and relax-ation) yielded no group differences (see Table 3.4).

**Therapy procedures**

*Massage therapy.* The massage therapy was given by a profes-sional massage therapist (different therapists each day) for 15 minutes a day, 2 days a week for 5 weeks, and the sessions were scheduled at noon each day. The subjects were seated fully

**Table 3.4** Means for demographic variables for massage therapy and relaxation control group measures (Study 4)

| Measures | Massage | Control | p |
|---|---|---|---|
| Age | 26.4 | 26.2 | NS |
| Gender (% female) | 79.5 | 80.2 | NS |
| Graduate degree (%) | 26.8 | 28.0 | NS |
| Income > $30 000 (%) | 7.8 | 9.1 | NS |
| Regular exercise (%) | 47.3 | 45.4 | NS |
| Tried relaxation (%) | 49.2 | 51.0 | NS |
| Tried massage (%) | 64.1 | 60.9 | NS |

clothed in a special massage chair (Fig. 3.1), and they were given a moderate pressure massage that was focused on the kneading of muscles.

1. *Back*:
   (a) compression to the back parallel to the spine from the shoulders to the base of the spine
   (b) compression to the entire back, adding some rocking
   (c) trapezius squeeze
   (d) finger pressure around scapula and shoulder
   (e) finger pressure along the length of the spine and back
   (f) circular strokes to the hips below the iliac crest

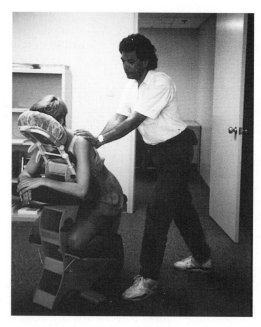

**Figure 3.1** Special massage chair.

2. *arms*:
   (a) dropping arms to the side; kneading arms from shoulders to lower arms
   (b) pressing down points on upper and lower arms
3. *hands*:
   (a) massaging entire hands; traction to the fingers
   (b) pressing the fleshy part of the palm between the thumb and index finger for 15 to 20 seconds
   (c) traction of the arms both in lateral and superior directions (arm in line with the body)
4. *neck*:
   (a) kneading cervical vertebrae
   (b) finger pressure along base of skull and along side of neck; pressing down on trapezius, finger pressure and squeezing continuing down the arms.

*Relaxation control group.* The subjects were asked to relax by tightening and relaxing the same body parts as those that were massaged for the massage therapy group (and in the same sequence). The subjects were briefly shown by a research assistant how to tighten and release their muscles which they were told would help them relax. This group was included as a control for focusing on the body and for standardizing activity level during the assessment sessions (controlling for movement artifact in the EEG measure).

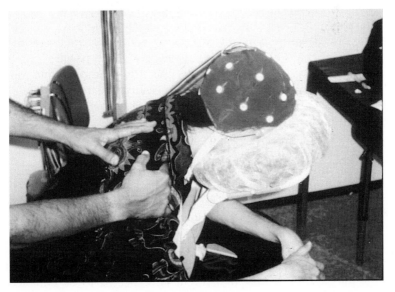

**Figure 3.2**   Subject wearing EEG cap while receiving massage.

**Assessment procedures** On the first and last day of the study the procedure was conducted in the following order for each subject.

1. The EEG cap was positioned on the subject's head (Fig. 3.2).
2. A saliva sample was taken for cortisol.
3. The subject completed the three long-term measures: the Life Events, Job Stress, and Chronic POMS Depression Scales.
4. The subject completed the session baseline measures: the POMS Depression, State Anxiety, and a math computation problem.
5. Immediately after the 15-minute massage/cortisol sessions the subject completed another math computation, the POMS Depression and State Anxiety Scale, and about 20 minutes after the end of the massage they provided another saliva sample for cortisol.

*Pre/post-therapy-session measures on first and last day.* The following measures were used to assess the immediate effects of the massage on the first and last days of the study.

• *The Profile of Mood States* (POMS) (McNair, Lorr & Droppleman 1971). This scale was used because positive mood state would be expected to affect alertness and performance on math computations and because massage therapy has been noted to improve mood state in stressed adolescents (Field et al 1992).

• *The STAI* (Spielberger, Gorsuch & Lushene 1970). This measure was included because state anxiety is known to negatively affect alertness and performance on cognitive tasks and because state anxiety typically decreases following massage therapy (Field et al 1992, Ironson et al 1996).

• *Salivary cortisol* (Appendix 2A). Saliva samples were collected and assayed for cortisol as a measure of stress that might be expected to affect alertness and performance on math computations. In addition, salivary cortisol levels decreased in at least two previous massage therapy studies (Field et al 1992, Ironson et al 1996). The samples were collected at the beginning of the therapy sessions and 20 minutes after the end of the sessions on the assessment days.

• *Math computations.* Before the massage sessions a series of 7 numbers was given, and after the massage a different series was given, and the subject was asked to add them. The time to complete the series and the correct/incorrect answers were recorded. This measure was used to determine the immediate effects of massage on a task that might be expected to be enhanced by alertness.

• *EEG procedure* (Appendix 3B). EEG was considered the primary dependent variable in this study as the physiological measure of alertness. Although subjects have anecdotally reported heightened alertness in previous studies, no direct measures have been made of alertness. Although EEG alpha and beta were noted to decrease (suggesting heightened alertness) in a previous study (Jodo et al 1988), face massage was used and no self-report or performance measures were included. EEG was recorded in the present study for 3-minute periods prior to, during, and after the therapy sessions with the subjects' eyes closed.

*First-day/last-day measures.* These longer-term measures were as follows.

• *Life Events Questionnaire.* (Appendix 3C). The Life Events Questionnaire is comprised of a list of 9 stressful events (e.g., death of mate or lover, major financial difficulties). The subject is asked to check which events have occurred in the last 4 weeks. The subject is then asked to rate how each event has affected his/her life, from not at all to very stressful on a 4 point scale. This measure was included to ensure that the results of this study were not negatively affected by significant life events.

• *Job Stress Yesterday Questionnaire* (Appendix 3D). This questionnaire measures job stress experienced yesterday and consists of 31 words or phrases requiring two responses each. The first response is a word or phrase describing the job (e.g. hectic, hassled, comfortable, too little time to think or plan). Possible answers are YES, NO or ? (cannot decide). If the phrase does describe the job yesterday, the subject is then asked to rate on a 4-point scale how much it bothers him/her. This questionnaire was included as a self-report measure on job stress.

## Results

**Self-report data** The analyses revealed the following (see Table 3.5).

1. The massage and relaxation control groups had significantly lower POMS depressed mood state scores following the first and last day sessions.

2. The massage therapy group had significantly lower state anxiety scores after the first and the last day sessions than the control group.

3. No group differences or time changes were noted for the Life Events Scale.

4. For the Job Stress Scale a significant repeated measures by group interaction effect was noted. A decrease in job stress was noted only for the massage group.

5. Both groups showed a decrease in chronic depressed mood state.

6. A *decrease* in salivary cortisol levels occurred on the first day for the massage group and an *increase* on the last day for the relaxation control group.

7. Massage also facilitated performance on math computation tasks (see Table 3.5). The massage therapy group performed better following the sessions on both the first and last days. The decreased time required to complete the math computation task was significantly greater for the massage therapy group, and the decrease in the number of errors was significantly greater for the massage therapy versus the control group

8. On the EEG data, delta, theta and alpha waves changed in the direction of heightened alertness for the massage therapy group (see Table 3.6).

**Table 3.5**  Means for massage therapy and relaxation control group measures (SDs in parentheses) (Study 4)

| Measures | Massage Day 1 Pre | Massage Day 1 Post | Massage Day 10 Pre | Massage Day 10 Post | Control Day 1 Pre | Control Day 1 Post | Control Day 10 Pre | Control Day 10 Post | Effects[1] |
|---|---|---|---|---|---|---|---|---|---|
| POMS depression | $1.5_a$ | $0.6_b$*** | $1.4_a$ | $0.5_b$*** | $2.1_a$ | $0.9_b$*** | $1.7_a$ | $0.8_b$** | S |
|  | (0.4) | (0.2) | (0.4) | (0.3) | (0.6) | (0.3) | (0.5) | (0.3) |  |
| State anxiety | $37.0_a$ | $30.0_b$**** | $38.5_a$ | $31.3_b$**** | $38.0_a$ | $37.0_a$ | $37.0_a$ | $5.2_a$ | SxG |
|  | (11.3) | (9.6) | (12.7) | (10.5) | (13.2) | (12.9) | (13.9) | (11.4) |  |
| Computation accuracy | $69.2_a$ | $89.2_b$** | $83.1_b$ | $96.2_c$** | $60.0_a$ | $68.2_a$ | $70.8_a$ | $72.3_a$ | SxG |
|  | (20.9) | (28.3) | (29.7) | (31.0) | (24.0) | (20.7) | (26.3) | (25.9) |  |
| Computation time | $250.0_a$ | $234.0_b$** | $232.5_b$ | $210.9_c$* | $249.0_a$ | $241.0_a$ | $231.1_b$ | $226.2_b$ | SxG |
|  | (85.1) | (72.3) | (75.9) | (64.0) | (82.6) | (71.8) | (65.0) | (62.3) |  |
| Salivary cortisol (ng) | $2.1_a$ | $1.6_b$** | $1.8_a$ | $2.0_a$ | $2.2_a$ | $2.0_a$ | $1.6_b$ | $2.1_a$*** | SxG |
|  | (0.5) | (0.5) | (0.4) | (0.5) | (0.7) | (0.6) | (0.4) | (0.6) |  |

| Measures | Massage Day 1 | | Massage Day 10 | | Control Day 1 | | Control Day 10 | | Effects |
|---|---|---|---|---|---|---|---|---|---|
| Life events | $8.0_a$ | | $7.4_a$ | | $9.5_a$ | | $8.9_a$ | | |
| Job stress[2] | $38.7_a$ | | $44.0_b$* | | $47.0_b$ | | $46.0_b$ | | PxG |
| Chronic POMs depression | $4.5_a$ | | $3.8_b$* | | $5.1_a$ | | $3.6_b$* | | P |

[1] G = group (massage/control); S = session (pre-session/post-session); P= phase (pre-treatment/post-treatment).
[2] Higher score is optimal.
* $p < 0.05$; ** $p < 0.01$; *** $p < 0.005$; **** $p < 0.001$.

**Table 3.6** Means of natural log of raw power for EEG delta, theta, alpha, and beta (SDs in parentheses) (Study 4)

| | | | **delta (1–4 Hz)** | | | |
| | Massage | | | | Control | |
| Pre | During | Post | | Pre | During | Post |
| --- | --- | --- | --- | --- | --- | --- |
| 4.29 | 4.55 | 4.16 | | 3.93 | 4.66 | 3.99 |
| (0.93) | (1.14) | (0.81) | | (0.96) | (1.34) | (1.22) |

Pre vs Dur vs Post: Trial $F = 6.32$ $p = 0.004$     Pre vs Dur: Trial $F = 8.07$ $p = 0.009$

| | | | **theta (5–7 Hz)** | | | |
| | Massage | | | | Control | |
| Pre | During | Post | | Pre | During | Post |
| --- | --- | --- | --- | --- | --- | --- |
| 3.02 | 2.71 | 3.02 | | 2.92 | 3.25 | 3.00 |
| (1.38) | (1.20) | (1.32) | | (1.58) | (1.26) | (1.45) |

| | | | **alpha (8–12 Hz)** | | | |
| | Massage | | | | Control | |
| Pre | During | Post | | Pre | During | Post |
| --- | --- | --- | --- | --- | --- | --- |
| 5.50 | 4.64 | 5.20 | | 4.99 | 4.87 | 5.61 |
| (1.58) | (1.30) | (1.67) | | (1.01) | (1.41) | (1.32) |

Pre vs Dur vs Post: Trial $F = 6.51$ $p = 0.003$     Group by Trial $F = 3.40$ $p = 0.04$
Pre vs Dur: Trial $F = 6.86$ $p = 0.02$     Pre vs Post: Group by Trial $F = 6.36$ $p = 0.02$

| | | | **beta (13–30 Hz)** | | | |
| | Massage | | | | Control | |
| Pre | During | Post | | Pre | During | Post |
| --- | --- | --- | --- | --- | --- | --- |
| 1.71 | 1.45 | 1.41 | | 2.03 | 3.04 | 2.84 |
| (1.81) | (2.14) | (1.95) | | (1.50) | (1.44) | (1.49) |

Pre vs Dur vs Post: Trial $F = 8.23$ $p = 0.001$     Group by Trial $F = 12.37$ $p = 0.000$
Pre vs Dur: Trial $F = 7.32$ $p = 0.01$     Group by Trial $F = 21.29$ $p = 0.000$
Pre vs Post: Trial $F = 13.68$ $p = 0.001$     Group by Trial $F = 5.20$ $p = 0.03$

## Discussion

These data, like those of other studies on massage therapy showed decreases in anxiety and stress hormones (cortisol) immediately after the sessions (Field et al 1992, Ironson et al 1996). And both the massage therapy and relaxation therapy groups showed increased delta activity, suggesting that they had both a relaxation effect and temporary and more chronic shifts in mood state which may have related to their relaxation. The decrease in self-reported depression is consistent with other massage studies (Field et al 1992, Ironson et al 1996) and other relaxation studies (Platania-Solazzo et al 1992).

The sessions in our study involved deep pressure in the head, neck, shoulders, and back regions. Surprisingly, instead of becoming sleepier after their midday massage, the participants reported experiencing heightened alertness, much like a runner's high. EEG recordings before, during and after the massage sessions confirmed the subjects' impressions. As compared with a group of relaxation therapy subjects, their levels of alpha wave activity significantly decreased during massage (in contrast to alpha levels typically increasing during sleep). This decrease, combined with increased delta and decreased beta waves, suggested a pattern of heightened alertness. We then added a math computation task to determine whether this EEG pattern of heightened alertness translated into performance. Following the massage sessions, computation time was significantly reduced and computation accuracy increased, showing that 15-minute massages during the lunch hour not only enhanced alertness, but also improved cognitive performance.

Heightened alertness and enhanced performance on math computations occurred in the massage therapy group. The massage sessions were characterized by an EEG pattern of alertness. Although delta increased for both groups of subjects, suggesting relaxation, the pattern of enhanced alertness (decreased alpha and decreased beta) occurred in the massage therapy group, while a pattern of drowsiness (increased alpha and increased beta) occurred in the relaxation control group. The decreased alpha and decreased beta were not surprising, since at least one other study documented EEG alpha decreases associated with facial massage (Jodo et al 1988). The correlation analysis further suggested that the accuracy of the math computations and the decrease in pre to during massage EEG alpha were related. Although the Alpha decrease occurred during the massages, it could have affected the state of alertness for enhancing accuracy after the massage. Further, the speed of performing the calculations and the decrease in EEG beta pre to post were related. This more contemporaneous relationship suggests that performance speed may have been related to decreased beta.

The superior performance of the massage therapy group might relate to the tactile and pressure stimulation. Tactile and pressure stimulation, in addition to enhancing the EEG patterns of alertness and math computations in this study, have been noted to enhance parasympathetic activity (elevated vagal tone) which is noted to be a more relaxed, alert state during which cognitive performance improves (Field et al 1992). Future research might add other measures such as vagal activity and catecholamines to further understand the underlying mechanism for the relation-ship between massage therapy and enhanced alertness.

In addition, a longer-term follow-up would be important to assess the persistence of the effects. Presumably, like exercise, a steady dose of massage may be required. Larger doses may also be more effective and result in more clinically meaningful changes in mood state and cortisol than occurred in this study. Finally, the cost-effectiveness of massage therapy would need to be documented for more widespread acceptance and adoption of the treatment.

## Study 5: Aromatherapy positively affects mood, EEG patterns of alertness, and math computations

Aromas have been used throughout history for their medicinal and mood-altering properties. Aroma molecules have direct effects on human behavior and physiology ranging from activation of memories to changes in mood or emotional states. Although much of what we know about these effects comes from anecdotal rather than empirical evidence (Buchbauer et al 1993, Tisserand 1989), these effects may be explained by the close association between the olfactory and limbic systems (Bear, Connors & Paradiso 1996).

Aromatherapy has been rapidly gaining popularity. The essential oils involved in aromatherapy are highly concentrated essences extracted from plants through the process of distillation. Each oil is said to produce a predictable and reproducible effect on the user when its fragrance is inhaled (Sanderson & Ruddle 1992, Tisserand 1989). For example in one study certain essential oils (lavender, spiced apple, and eucalyptus) modified EEG activity, including increasing relaxation as suggested by increases in alpha power (Lorig and Schwartz 1987). In another study Lorig and colleagues found that frontal beta EEG activity increased during lavender and decreased during spiced apple presentation (Lorig et al 1990). Parasuraman and his colleagues (1992) found that subjects exposed to a peppermint aroma were better able to sustain attention as assessed by an increase in skin conductance levels and sustained event-related potential across the attention task. Other studies have supported these EEG findings. For example Badia and colleagues recorded high-frequency bursts in the EEG of subjects who were presented with a peppermint aroma during sleep (Badia et al 1990). Aromatherapy research has also shown behavioral changes including improved mood following presentation of chamomile oil (Roberts & Williams 1992), positive affect while smelling vanillin (Miltner, Matjak, Diekmann & Brody 1994), enhanced attention and performance on visual vigilance tasks following presentation of peppermint aroma (Warm et al 1991), and decreased anxiety and tension following lavender, spiced apple, or eucalyptus aroma presentation (Lorig & Schwartz 1987).

This study examined aromatherapy effects on anxiety, mood, alertness, EEG activity and math computations (Diego 1998). Two aromas were examined: an alerting odor (rosemary) and a relaxing odor (lavender). After the aromatherapy session the subjects who experienced the lavender aroma were expected to report less anxiety, better mood, and to show an increase in EEG power in the alpha and beta bands, suggesting increased relaxation. In contrast, subjects who were presented the rosemary aroma were expected to show greater alertness as suggested by decreased alpha and beta power and better performance on the math computations. In addition the cortisol levels were expected to decrease for both groups as they have in other relaxation studies. For example, in a previous EEG study subjects who were given massage therapy (1) showed a decrease in frontal alpha and beta power (suggesting alertness), (2) showed an increase in frontal delta power (suggesting relaxation), (3) reported feeling better, and (4) performed better on math computations (Field, Ironson et al 1996).

### Method

**Sample** The subjects were 40 faculty and staff members of the University of Miami Medical School (30 females, 10 males, mean age = 30.9). They were middle to upper middle socioeconomic status (mean = 2.7 on the Hollingshead) and were 43% white, 15% African American, and 42% Hispanic. The participants were randomly assigned to the lavender or rosemary aroma conditions. The groups did not differ on the above demographic variables.

**Aromatherapy procedure** The aromatherapy was given by a research assistant to subjects seated in a special massage chair. Three drops of lavender or rosemary essential oil diluted to 10% concentration in grapeseed oil (provided by Aromatherapy Associates, Inc.) were placed on a cotton dental swab and presented in a 100 mL plastic vial which the subjects held about 3 inches from their nose for a period of 3 minutes. Subjects were instructed to breathe normally through their noses and sit quietly with their eyes closed.

**Assessment** The assessments were conducted in the following order.

1. the *EEG cap* was positioned on the subject's head.
2. A *saliva sample* was taken for cortisol.
3. The subject completed the session baseline measures, including the *demographic questionnaire*, the *STAI* (Spielberger et al 1970), the *Profile of Mood States* (POMS) (McNair et al 1971), the *tense–relaxed and drowsy–alert visual analogue mood scales*, and the *math computations*.
4. Then the *aromatherapy* was given.
5. Immediately after the aromatherapy, the subject completed another math computation, the POMS depression scale, and the STAI to assess anxiety.
6. About 20 minutes after the end of the aroma session the subject provided another saliva sample for cortisol.

Pre–post measures included:

1. the POMS (McNair et al 1971)
2. the STAI (Spielberger et al 1970)
3. two visual analogue scales (tense–relaxed and drowsy–alert) on which the subjects circled the number (on a 10-point ordinal scale) corresponding to the way they felt at that moment. On the tense–relaxed scale, a score of 0 was assigned to feeling 'very tense' and a score of 10 to being 'very relaxed'. On the drowsy–alert scale a score of 0 was assigned to feeling 'very drowsy' and a score of 10 to feeling 'very alert'
4. *saliva samples* which were collected and assayed for cortisol as a measure of stress that might be expected to affect alertness and performance on math computations (Appendix 2A)
5. *math computations* involving averaging a series of seven single-digit numbers. The time needed to complete the computation and the accuracy of the response was recorded. This measure was used to determine whether the alerting effects attributed to rosemary would translate into superior performance
6. *the EEG procedure*, which was considered the primary dependent variable in this study as the physiological measure of relaxation and alertness. EEG was recorded for 3-minute periods prior to, during and after the therapy sessions, with the subjects' eyes closed.

## Results

Data analyses revealed the following (Table 3.7).

1. There was a significant decrease in the State Anxiety scores of both groups.

2. Only the lavender group had significantly better mood (lower POMS scores) after the aroma session.

3. Both groups were feeling more relaxed.

4. The rosemary group reported feeling more alert.

5. Both groups completed the math computations faster (Table 3.8), but only the lavender group's accuracy improved.

6. Alpha power significantly increased after lavender, suggesting increased drowsiness, while alpha power decreased from pre to during and pre to post after the rosemary, suggesting increased alertness. Beta power increased for lavender, suggesting decreased alertness, and decreased for rosemary, suggesting increased alertness.

## Discussion

The present study evaluated the effects of two commonly used aromas which affected anxiety, mood, relaxation, alertness, math computations, and EEG activity. Our findings support other research studies showing that certain aromas can positively influence mood (Roberts & Williams 1992). The lavender group reporting feeling more relaxed, and their increase in beta power supports previous findings on lavender's ability to increase frontal beta power (Lorig et al 1990), promote drowsiness (Buchbauer et al 1991), and induce sleep (van Toller 1988). Those who were exposed to the rosemary aroma showed increased alertness both by their self report and the decreases noted in alpha and beta

**Table 3.7** Means for lavender and rosemary group measures (SDs in parentheses) (Study 5)

| Measure | Lavender (N = 20) | | Rosemary (N = 20) | | Effects |
|---|---|---|---|---|---|
| | Pre | Post | Pre | Post | |
| State Anxiety[1] | 34.32$_a$ (9.53) | 31.21$_b$ (8.75) | 33.30$_a$ (9.33) | 26.30$_b$ (5.91) | T* |
| Depressed mood[1] | 2.66$_a$ (2.63) | 1.16$_b$ (1.64) | 1.45$_b$ (3.05) | 1.74$_b$ (3.73) | G x T** T† |
| Tense–relaxed | 6.10$_a$ (2.47) | 7.68$_b$ (2.02) | 7.00$_a$ (2.39) | 8.70$_b$ (1.34) | T**** |
| Drowsy–alert | 6.16$_a$ (2.91) | 5.95$_a$ (2.71) | 6.00$_a$ (2.34) | 7.30$_b$ (1.62) | G x T† |
| Computation time[1] | 5.14$_a$ (1.80) | 4.49$_b$ (1.94) | 5.23$_a$ (1.75) | 4.52$_b$ (1.26) | T*** |
| Computation accuracy | 2.55$_a$ (1.79) | 3.10$_b$ (1.59) | 2.25$_a$ (1.83) | 2.50$_a$ (1.64) | T* |

[1] Lower is optimal.
† $p < 0.1$; * $p < 0.05$; ** $p < 0.01$; *** $p < 0.005$; **** $p < 0.001$.
Different subscript letters denote significant differences.

**Table 3.8**   Group by trial by region effects for frontal and parietal EEG log power values (SDs in parentheses) (Study 5)

| | alpha (8–12 Hz) | | |
|---|---|---|---|
| Lavender | $3.07_a$ (3.47) | $3.40_a$ (2.90) | $3.72_b{}^\dagger$ (2.74) |
| Rosemary | $4.16_a$ (2.22) | 3.74b** (2.15) | $3.72_c{}^\dagger$ (2.41) |

Group x Time $F$ (1.37) = 2.588, $p$ = 0.089;    Region $F$ (1.37) = 119.71, $p$ = 0.000.

| | beta 1 (13–20 Hz) | | |
|---|---|---|---|
| Lavender | 0.57 (3.35) | 0.79 (2.77) | 0.96 (2.67) |
| Rosemary | $1.07_a$ (2.05) | $0.96_b{}^\dagger$ (1.99) | $1.14_a$ (2.11) |

Region x Time $F$ (1.37) = 4.772, $p$ = 0.015;    Region $F$ (1.37) = 30.38, $p$ < 0.000.

| | beta 2 (21–30 Hz) | | |
|---|---|---|---|
| Lavender | $-0.17_a$ (3.16) | $0.06_a$ (2.58) | $0.27_b$** (2.53) |
| Rosemary | $0.53_a$ (1.76) | $0.47_a$ (1.87) | $0.80_b{}^\dagger$ (2.14) |

Time $F$ (1.37) = 6.565, $p$ = 0.004.

$\dagger$ $p < 0.1$; * $p < 0.05$; ** $p < 0.01$.
Different subscript letters denote significant differences.

power. These findings support the belief that rosemary is an alerting aroma (van Toller 1988).

The math computation results suggest that, although both groups performed the computations faster after the aroma session, only the lavender group showed improved accuracy on math computations following the sessions. This finding was surprising because the lavender group did not show the enhanced alertness EEG pattern that the rosemary group showed. Perhaps as reflected in both self report and EEG data the lavender group was more relaxed and thus better able to concentrate. This and previous research indicate that aromas can effect psychological and physiological changes. Further research is needed on the underlying mechanisms of these effects.

These EEG pattern changes might explain the enhanced attentiveness noted in all of the studies. Other alternative or parallel mechanisms could include increased vagal activity or increased dopamine. Several variables such as these would need to be included in mechanism studies on facilitating attentiveness by massage therapy. All of the above mechanisms have been hypothesized for the positive effects of massage on depressive disorders. Enhanced dopamine is a likely candidate, particularly since the publication of the depression model suggesting elevated norepinephrine and depleted dopamine in depressed animals (Weiss et al 1997) and our own data showing the same patterns in humans and the decrease in norepinephrine and increase in dopamine levels following massage in depressed adolescents (Field, Grizzle, et al 1996).

REFERENCES

American Psychiatric Association 1987 Diagnostic and statistical manual for mental disorders, 3rd edn, revised. APA, Washington, DC

Anderson JC, Williams S, McGee R et al 1987 DSM-III disorders in preadolescent children: prevalence in a large sample from the general population. Archives of General Psychiatry 44:69–76

Badia P, Wesensten N, Lammers W, Culpepper J, Harsh J 1990 Responsiveness to olfactory stimuli presented in sleep. Physiology & Behavior 48:87–90

Barkley RA 1989 Attention deficit hyperactivity disorder. In: Mash EJ, Barkley RA (eds) Treatment of childhood disorders. Guilford Press, New York, pp 39–72

Bear MF, Connors BW, Paradiso MA 1996 Neuroscience: exploring the brain. Williams & Wilkins, Baltimore

Biederman J, Newcorn J, Spirch S 1991 Comorbidity of attention deficit hyperactivity disorder with conduct, depressive, anxiety, and other disorders. American Journal of Psychiatry 148:564–577

Blakemore B, Shindler S, Conte R 1993 A problem solving training program for parents of children with attention deficit hyperactivity disorder. Canadian Journal of School Psychology 9 (1):65–85

Brown DD, Mucci WG, Hetzler RK, Knowlton RG 1989 Cardiovascular and ventilatory responses during formalized Tai Chi Chuan exercise. Research Quarterly Exercise Sport 60:246–250

Brown DR, Wang Y, Ward A, Ebbeling CB, Fortlage L, Puleo E, Benson H, Rippe JM 1995 Chronic psychological effects of exercise and exercise plus cognitive strategies. Medical Science Sports Exercise 27(5):765–775

Bryant BK 1982 An index of empathy for children and adolescents. Child Development 53:413–425

Buchbauer B, Jirovetz L, Jager W, Dietrich H, Plank C, Karamat E 1991 Aromatherapy: evidence for sedative effects of the essential oils of lavender after inhalation. Naturforschung 46:1067–1072

Buchbauer G, Jirovetz L, Jager W, Plank C, Dietrich H 1993 Fragrance compounds and essential oils with sedative effects upon inhalation. Journal of Pharmaceutical Sciences 82:660–664

Conners CK 1985 The Conners rating scales: instruments for the assessment of childhood psychopathology. Unpublished manuscript, Children's Hospital National Medical Center, Washington DC

Damico SK, Armstrong MB 1996 Intervention strategies for students with ADHD: creating a holistic approach. Seminars in Speech & Language 17 (1):21–34

Diego M, Jones NA, Field T et al 1998 Aromatherapy reduces anxiety and enhances EEG patterns associated with positive mood and alertness. International Journal of Neuroscience 96:217–224

Evans RW, Gualtieri CT, Hicks RE 1986 Substrate for stimulant drug effects in hyperactive children. Clinical Neuropharmacology 9:264–281

Field T 1990 Newborn behavior, vagal tone and catecholamine activity in cocaine exposed infants. Symposium presented at the International Society of Infant Studies, Montreal, Canada, April 1990

Field T, Grizzle N, Scafidi F & Schanberg S 1996 Massage and relaxation therapies' effect on depressed adolescent mothers. Adolescence 31:903–911

Field T, Morrow C, Valdeon C, Larson S, Kuhn C, Schanberg S 1992 Massage therapy reduces anxiety in child and adolescent psychiatric patients. Journal of the American Academy of Child and Adolescent Psychiatry 31:135–131

Field T, Ironson G, Scafidi F, Nawrocki T, Goncalves A, Burman I, Pickens J, Fox N, Schanberg S, Kuhn C 1996 Massage therapy reduces anxiety and enhances EEG pattern of alertness and math computations. International Journal of Neuroscience 86:197–205

Field T, Lasko D, Mundy P, Henteleff T, Talpins S, Dowling M 1996 Autistic children's attentiveness and responsivity improved after touch therapy. Journal of Autism & Developmental Disorder 27 (3):329–334

Field T, Seligman S, Scafidi S, Schanberg S 1996 Alleviating posttraumatic stress in children following Hurricane Andrew. Journal of Applied Developmental Psychology 17:37–50

Field T, Quintino O, Hernandez-Reif M 1998 Adolescents with attention deficit hyperactivity disorder benefit from massage therapy. Adolescence 33:103–108

Goyette CH, Conners CK, Ulrich RF 1978 Normative data on Revised Conners Parent and Teachers Rating Scales. Journal of Abnormal Child Psychology 6:221–236

Handen BL, Feldman H, Gosling A et al 1991 Adverse side effects of methylphenidate among mentally retarded children with ADHD. Journal of the American Academy of Child and Adolescent Psychiatry 30:241–245

Hsu L, Wang S, Kappagoda CT 1985 Effect of Tai Chi Chua on the response to the treadmill exercise. In: Beamish RE, Singal PK, Dhalla NS (eds) Stress and heart disease Martinus Nijhoff, Boston

Iaboni F, Douglas V, Ditto B 1997 Psychophysiological response of ADHD children to reward and extinction. Psychophysiology 34(1):116–123

Ironson G, Field T, Scafidi F, Hashimoto M, Kumar M, Kumar A, Price A, Goncalves A, Burman I, Tetenman I 1996 Massage therapy is associated with enhancement of the immune system's cytotoxic capacity. International Journal of Neuroscience 84:205–217

Ivancevitch JM, Matteson MT, Freedman SM, Phillips JS 1990 Worksite stress management interventions. American Psychologist 45:252–261

Jin P 1989 Changes in heart rate, noradrenaline, cortisol and mood during Tai Chi. Journal of Psychosomatic Research 33(2) 197–206

Jin P 1992 Efficacy of Tai Chi, brisk walking, meditation and reading in reducing mental and emotional stress. Journal of Psychosomatic Research 36:361–370

Jodo E, Yamada, Y, Hatayama, T, Abe T, Maruyama 1988 Effects of facial massage on the spontaneous EEG. Tohoku Psycologica Folia 47:8–15

Jones NA, Field T, Davalos M, Pickens J 1997 Brain electrical activity stability in infants/children of depressed mothers. Child Psychiatry and Human Development 28(2):175–186

Krug D, Arick, J, Almond P 1979 Autism screening instrument for educational planning: background and development. In: Gilliam J (ed), Autism: diagnosis, instruction, management and research. University of Texas Press, Austin,

Lorig TS, Schwartz GE 1987 EEG activity during fine fragrance administration. Psychophysiology 24:599

Lorig TS, Schwartz GE 1998 EEG activity during relaxation and food imagery. Imagination, Cognition & Personality 8:201–208

Lorig TS, Herman KB, Schwartz GE, Cain WS 1990 EEG activity during administration of low-concentration odors. Bulletin of the Psychonomic Society 28:405–408

McNair DM, Lorr M 1964 An analysis of mood in neurotics. Journal of Abnormal Social Psychology 69:620–627

McNair DM, Lorr M, Droppleman LF 1971 Profile of mood states. Educational and Industrial Testing Service, San Diego

Mehrabian A, Epstein N 1972 A measure of emotional empathy. Journal of Personality, 40, 525–543

Miltner W, Matjak M, Diekmann H, Brody S 1994 Emotional qualities of odors and their influence on the startle reflex in humans. Psychophysiology 31:107–110

Mundy P, Sigman M, Kasari C 1994 Joint attention, developmental level, and symptom presentation in autism. Development and Psychopathology 6:389–401

Parasuraman R, Warm JS, Dember WN 1992 Effects of olfactory stimulation on skin conductance and event-related brain potentials during visual sustained attention. New York, Fragrance Research Fund

Parraga HC, Cochran MK 1992 Emergence of motor and vocal tics during imipramine administration in two children. Journal of Child and Adolescent Psychopharmacology 2:227–234

Platania-Solazzo A, Field T, Blank J, Seligman F, Kuhn C, Schanberg S, Saab P 1992 Relaxation therapy reduces anxiety in child/adolescent psychiatry patients. Acta Paedopsychiatrica 55:115–120

Porges SW 1991 Vagal tone: a mediator of affect. In: Garber JA Dodge KA (eds) The development of affect regulation and dysregulation. Cambridge University Press, New York, pp 111–128

Pugtach D, Haskell D, McNair DM 1969 Predictors and patterns of change associated with the course of time limited psychotherapy. Mimeo Report

Radloff L 1977 The CES-D scale: a self-report depression scale for research in the general population. Applied Psychological Measures 1:385–401

Roberts A, Williams JMG 1992 The effect of olfactory stimulation on fluency, vividness of imagery and associated mood: a preliminary study. British Journal of Medical Psychology 65:197–199

Rogeness GA, Javors MA, Pliszka SR 1992 Neurochemistry and child adolescent psychiatry. Journal of the American Academy of Child and Adolescent Psychiatry 31:765–781

Sanderson H, Ruddle J 1992 Aromatherapy and occupational therapy. British Journal of Occupational Therapy 55:310–314

Schachar R, Tannock R 1983 Childhood hyperactivity and psychostimulants: a review of extended treatment studies. Journal of the American Medical Association 260:2256–2258

Schwiebert V, Sealander K, Tollerud T 1995 Attention-deficit hyperactivity disorder: an overview for school counselors. Elementary School Guidance Counseling 29:249–259

Seibert JM, Hogan AE, Mundy PC 1982 Assessing interactional competencies: the Early Social-Communication Scales. Infant Mental Health Journal 3:244–245

Spielberger CD 1972 Anxiety as an emotional state. In: Spielberger CD (ed.) Anxiety: current trends in theory and research. Academic Press, New York

Spielberger CD, Gorsuch RL, Lushene RE 1970 The State Trait Anxiety Inventory Consulting Psychologists Press, Palo Alto, CA

Swanson JM, McBurnett K, Christian DL, Wigal T 1995 Stimulant medication and treatment of children with ADHD. In: Ollendick TH, Prinz RZ (eds) Advances in Clinical Child Psychology 17:265–322

Tisserand R 1989 The practice of aromatherapy. CW Daniel, Saffron Walden

van Toller S 1988 Emotion and the brain. In: van Toller S, Dodd GH (eds) Perfumery: the psychology and biology of fragrance Chapman and Hall, London

Warm JS, Dember WN, Parasuraman R 1991 Effects of olfactory stimulation on performance and stress in a visual sustained attention task. Journal of the Society of Cosmetic Chemists 42:199–210

Weiss JM, Bonsall RW, Demetrikopoulos MK, Emery MS, West CHK 1997 Galanin: a significant role in depression? Annals of the New York Academy of Sciences 863:364–382

Wolf SL, Barnhart HX, Kutner NG, McNeely E, Coogler C, Xue T 1996 Reducing frailty and falls in older persons: an investigation of Tai Chi and computerized balance training. Atlanta FICSIT Group. Frailty and injuries: cooperative studies on intervention techniques. Journal of the American Geriatrics Society 44(5):489–497

# Alleviating depression and anxiety

We review in this chapter studies using massage therapy with reactive depressions, such as post-traumatic stress disorder, and more chronic depressive disorders, including chronic fatigue and bulimia. These disorders typically feature depression and anxiety as well as hormonal and neurotransmitter imbalances. As already noted, massage therapy has effectively reduced these imbalances in pain syndromes, suggesting that this kind of therapy might also be effective with depression and anxiety.

## POST-TRAUMATIC STRESS IN CHILDREN

### Study 1: Alleviating post-traumatic stress in children following Hurricane Andrew

Recent studies have described a number of post-trauma responses in children that are similar to those described for adults and for the diagnosis of post-traumatic stress disorder in the DSM-III (Newman 1976, Pynoos & Eth 1985, Terr 1979). Typically these symptoms are observed following natural disasters or human-induced disasters.

Symptoms frequently described for the children include numbing of responsiveness (Frederick 1985, Green 1983, Pynoos & Eth 1985), increased arousal (Bloch, Silber & Perry 1956, Burke et al 1982), and conduct problems that persist for several months following the traumatic event. In a study by Pynoos et al (1987), for example, post-traumatic stress disorder (PTSD) was noted in as many as 60% of children after a fatal sniper attack on their elementary school playground. Children with the most severe initial reaction continued to show high levels of PTSD symptomatology 14 months later (Nader et al 1990).

At least one hurricane has been studied for its effects on children (Lonigan et al 1991). Self-report data collected about 3 months after Hurricane Hugo suggested that the children who experienced the more severe exposure to the hurricane had significantly higher anxiety scores and significantly more PTSD symptoms. In a subsequent study, parents of 200 preschool children were asked to observe their children's play and verbalizations in the year following Hurricane Hugo (Saylor, Swenson & Powell 1992). One of the most frequent activities was re-enactment and discussion of the traumatic event during play. This observation has been made in other natural disasters such as the Aberfan mine collapse and land slide (Lacey 1972), an Italian earthquake (Galante & Foa 1986), a tornado in Mississippi (Bloch et al 1956), and an Australian bush fire (McFarlane 1987).

Other treatment techniques suggested by Frederick (1985) include the coloring story book, drawings (structured and unstructured), play therapy and group psychotherapy by trained therapists, and a treatment called 'Incident-specific treatment'. This treatment involved returning the children to the location of the catastrophe either 'in vitro' by re-establishing the scene in the mind of the child or 'in vivo' by actually physically returning the child to the scene.

Another potential treatment strategy was suggested to us by the grade school teachers whose informal observations suggested a decrease in physical contact initiated by parents and teachers toward children after Hurricane Andrew. This decrease in physical contact was the teachers' most frequently reported change following the hurricane. The teachers suggested that the adults in these children's lives were experiencing post-traumatic stress symptoms themselves and were both preoccupied with those symptoms and not wanting to convey their tension to their children, which may have been the reason for their initiating less physical contact. Nonetheless, the children initiated more physical contact and showed excessive clinging behavior as if desiring more physical contact. These observations coupled with data from earlier studies on reducing stress in children led us to conduct a massage therapy intervention with grade school children following Hurricane Andrew.

The purpose of this study was to determine whether massage therapy might reduce the anxiety and depression levels of the children as measured by behavioral observations, the children's drawings and the children's cortisol levels. In a previous study on hospitalized children with depression and conduct disorder, five 30-minute massage therapy sessions led to reduced anxiety and depression symptoms, fewer self-reported symptoms, improved sleep patterns, and decreased cortisol levels (Field et al 1992). Parallels in the post-hurricane and hospitalized depressed and conduct disorder children include their anxiety, depression, and touch deprivation. We expected that massage therapy would lower the anxiety and depression levels and would decrease cortisol levels in the children experiencing post-traumatic stress following Hurricane Andrew, just as it had for the hospitalized children with psychiatric problems. Although the underlying mechanism for massage therapy reducing anxiety and depression is not clear, it probably relates to the reduction in stress hormones typically noted following massage therapy, including the reduction of norepinephrine and cortisol levels previously reported (Field et al 1992).

## Method

**Sample** The sample was comprised of 60 low to middle SES grade school age children (34 males, 26 females) in grades 1 to 5 (mean age = 7.5, mean grade = 2.2). The ethnicity of the children was representative of their school (48% Hispanic, 39% non-Hispanic White, and 13% Black). The children were randomly selected by the teachers (using a table of numbers) from a pool of children approximately twice the sample size who had been referred by the classroom teachers to the school counselors for classroom behavior problems following Hurricane Andrew. Four weeks after Hurricane Andrew, when we had completed a pilot study and when the school was back on its 'normal' routine, we recruited a sample of 60 children. They were randomly assigned (following informed parental consent and child assent) to a massage therapy or a video attention control group, and the sessions were started immediately.

**Measures** Twelve psychology graduate students (who were unaware of the children's group assignment) read the self-report scales to the children at the beginning and at the end of the study. Those measures given only at the beginning of the study included an Activity Check List (created for this study), a questionnaire on the details of the hurricane experience (also created for this study), and the Posttraumatic Stress Disorder Reaction Index (Frederick 1985). Measures given at both the beginning and end of the study included the Children's Manifest Anxiety Scale (Reynolds & Richmond 1985), the Center for Epidemiological Studies Depression Scale (Radloff 1977), a 'Drawing of Yourself' (Field & Reite 1984), and the Relaxation Rating made by the interviewer/observer. Measures given before and after the first and last therapy sessions (massage and video) were used to assess the immediate effects of the therapy. These included the State Anxiety Inventory for Children (STAIC) (Spielberger, Gorsuch & Lushene 1970), the Smiley Faces Scale, and assays of salivary cortisol levels. Initially we had also intended to solicit teacher and parent reports of child classroom and home behaviors, but during piloting we discovered very low levels of teacher and parent compliance during this stressful period. The baseline measures were taken on the first day of the study, and the follow-up measures were taken one day before the last treatment session. An additional session was scheduled after the outcome assessment session because the children in a previous study (both massage therapy and video control children) seemed to be showing separation anxiety symptoms during their last session, having apparently become attached to being in the study.

*Measures taken only at the beginning of the study*

1. *Activity Checklist.* This questionnaire was designed to assess group equivalence on demographic, social support and optimism measures. The questionnaire included classroom measures such as grades in school, popularity at school, number of close friends in and out of school, activity measures including number of after-school activities, important relationships other than family members, quantity and quality of conversations with mother, frequency of physical contact with mother, and the child's hopefulness about things improving.

2. *'What Happened to You During and After Hurricane Andrew' (Hurricane Impact) Questionnaire.* This questionnaire included 13 questions on events during the hurricane, and 16 questions on events after the hurricane, designed to assess group equivalence on hurricane impact. Examples of questions on events during the hurricane included:

- Did any windows or doors break or did your roof come off in the place you stayed while the hurricane was here?
- Did you get hurt during the hurricane?
- Was anyone with you very scared during the hurricane?

Examples of questions on events after the hurricane included:

- Will you have to move to a new place for a long time because of the hurricane?
- Did a grownup in your home lose his or her job because of the hurricane?
- Did you lose many things in your home because of the hurricane?

The children were considered a high exposure group if they responded positively on more than two items on each of these sets of questions. This criterion was based on a similar criterion used in adult disaster research.

3. *The PTSD Reaction Index* (Frederick 1985). The PTSD Reaction Index is based on the criteria for PTSD described in the DSM-III. Originally used for adults' reactions to traumatic events and incident-specific stress symptoms following those events, a revised version was designed with appropriate wording for school-aged children. The 20-item scale is scored as a 5-point Likert Index from 0 (none of the time) to 4 (most of the time). The items include:

- anxiety items (for example, 'I'm more jumpy or nervous than before')
- bad cognitions ('I have bad dreams since the hurricane')
- fears ('I feel afraid or upset with thoughts about the hurricane')
- attention problems ('I remember things well')
- vegetative signs ('I sleep well').

Children who report positive responses to 10–12 items are considered moderately stressed (a score greater than 25), children with a score greater than 40 are considered severely stressed, and those with a score greater than 60 are considered very severely stressed.

*Measures taken before the sessions at the beginning and end of the study*

1. *The Revised Children's Manifest Anxiety Scale* (Reynolds & Richmond 1985). This is a 37-item true/false self-report measure of trait anxiety.

2. *Self-drawings* (Field & Reite 1984). For these the child was given a blank sheet of paper and a set of colored magic markers and asked to make a drawing of self. The drawings were then scored for the following problems (1 point per problem):

(a) small figure on paper;
(b) dull colors;

(c) sad face;

(d) missing body parts;

(e) distorted body parts;

(f) displaced body parts. Self-drawings have been known to relate to other stress measures (e.g., the drawing score was significantly related to nightwakings in Field & Reite 1984)

3. *Relaxation level.* This is a visual analogue scale (0–100) on which an observer rates the child's apparent relaxation level.

*Measures taken before and after the massage/video sessions at beginning and end of the study*

1. *State Trait Anxiety Inventory for Children* (STAIC) (Spielberger et al 1973). The STAIC is an adaptation of the STAI specifically designed for the study of anxiety in school-age children. The inventory consists of 20 items. Characteristic items include 'I feel … very tense, tense or not tense', 'I feel … very nervous, nervous or not nervous', and 'I feel … very relaxed, relaxed or not relaxed.' Research has demonstrated that the STAIC-State scale is sensitive to stressful situations.

2. *Happy Face Scale* (Appendix 3A). Four 'faces' ranging from sad to neutral to partially happy (semi-grin) to happy (wide smile) are presented to the child. The child is then asked which face best describes the way he or she feels right now. The scales range from 1–4, with a higher number reflecting happier, more positive faces. This measure was used to assess the child's mood state before and after massage therapy/video control. We were interested in the sad/happy dimension, as opposed to other affects such as fear and anger, because the PTSD children often appeared sad, but rarely fearful or angry.

3. *Saliva cortisol.* (Appendix 2A) All sessions were held during the late mornings (because school was only in session during the mornings) thus enabling us to assay cortisol levels at the same time (controlling for diurnal variation) and at a time when cortisol levels are typically higher (cortisol being generally highest in the early morning and lowest in midafternoon).

**Massage therapy** The massage therapy group children received 30 minutes of back massage per session twice per week for 8 days over a 1-month period by a different volunteer massage therapy student for each session (10 therapists for 30 children). The massage entailed moderate pressure and smooth stroking movements for 5-minute periods in each of three regions: up and down the neck, from the neck across the shoulders and back to the neck, and from the neck to the waist and back to the neck along the vertebral column. The 15-minute sequence was comprised of 30 back-and-forth strokes per region at 10 seconds each. This same 15-minute sequence was repeated in its entirety for a total session of 30 minutes. The children were asked to remain still and quiet for the 30-minute session and told that the massage procedure would help them relax, and the massage therapist remained silent during the sessions.

**Video attention control group** The video attention control group was seen at the same time of day for a videotape viewing session for the same period of time (30 minutes per day twice per week for 8 days) as the massage therapy group. During this condition, the child simply sat and watched 'Milo and Otis' or 'Beauty and the Beast' with a psychology graduate student. The graduate student maintained physical contact by sitting the child on her lap or putting her arm around the child. The children were asked to remain still and quiet for the 30-minute session, and the graduate student remained silent. The children were told that the video procedure would help them relax. The pilot study data suggested that these films were relaxing for the children. This control condition was employed to ensure that any changes noted in behavior or physiology during the massage therapy sessions were not simply related to temporal or activity variation in these measures, to clinical improvement from other treatments, or from the physical presence and attention provided by the therapist. The same measurements and the same time frame as those used to assess the massage therapy group were also used to assess the video control group.

## Results

As can be seen in Table 4.1, the two groups of children did not differ on age, grade level, academic grades in school, number of friends, number of extracurricular activities and the presence of a close person (significant adult) in their lives. The groups had Hurricane Impact and PTSD Reaction Index scores in the severe range, and the groups did not differ on these measures.

**Table 4.1** Demographic variables (Study 1)

| | Groups | | |
|---|---|---|---|
| Variables | Massage therapy | Video control | $p$ |
| Age | 7.7 | 7.3 | NS |
| Grade level | 2.4 | 2.0 | NS |
| Academic grades | 2.7 | 3.2 | NS |
| # friends | 3.2 | 3.3 | NS |
| # extracurricular activities | 1.0 | 1.3 | NS |
| # close persons | 1.0 | 0.8 | NS |
| Hurricane Impact score | 3.6 | 3.6 | NS |
| PTSD Reaction Index score | 44.1 | 43.6 | NS |

**Immediate effects of treatment** As can be seen in Table 4.2, the following effects emerged:

1. The massage therapy versus the video control children reported less anxiety after the massage therapy session on both the first day and the last day, and they also showed a greater decrease from the first to the last day on state anxiety before the session.

2. For the *Happy Face Scale*, the children in the massage therapy versus the video control group showed a significant increase in their positive ratings from pre to post massage therapy on the first day and from pre to post massage therapy on the last day.

3. For *salivary cortisol* levels, the massage therapy versus the video control group showed a significant decrease from pre to post massage therapy on the first day and on the last day. A greater percentage of the massage therapy than video control group children showed lower levels of salivary cortisol on day 8 versus day 1.

**Beginning/end of study measures** As can be seen in Table 4.2, the following effects emerged:

1. the massage therapy versus the video control group children had lower *Children's Manifest Anxiety Scale* scores on the last day than the first day.

2. On the *CESD Depression Scale*, the massage therapy versus the video control group children showed a significant decrease over the period of the study.

**Table 4.2** Treatment effects (Study 1)

| Variables | Massage therapy | | | | Video control | | | |
|---|---|---|---|---|---|---|---|---|
| | First day | | Last day | | First day | | Last day | |
| | Pre | Post | Pre | Post | Pre | Post | Pre | Post |
| *Immediate effects* | | | | | | | | |
| State Anxiety | 35.5 | 30.6** | 33.0* | 28.7**** | 36.7 | 34.5 | 35.0 | 33.8 |
| Smiley Face | 3.4 | 4.0*** | 3.7* | 4.0** | 3.3 | 3.5 | 3.6 | 3.7 |
| Saliva cortisol (ng/mL) | 1.9 | 1.2*** | 1.7 | 1.3* | 1.9 | 1.7 | 1.6 | 2.0 |
| *Long-term effects* | | First day | | Last day | | First day | | Last day |
| Children's Manifest Anxiety | | 17.0 | | 12.3*** | | 16.6 | | 15.9 |
| CESD (Depression) | | 26.0 | | 16.0**** | | 25.6 | | 27.1 |
| Drawing score | | 3.6 | | 2.8* | | 3.9 | | 4.0 |
| Relaxation level | | 47.4 | | 81.9** | | 43.3 | | 49.1 |

Note: For immediate effects, asterisks after post means are pre–post session comparisons. Asterisks after pre means last day (day 8) are for comparisons between day 1 and day 8 baseline (pre) means. For the long-term effects, rows on the bottom half of the table, asterisks after last day are for comparisons between day 1 and day 8.
* $p < 0.05$; ** $p < 0.01$; *** $p < 0.005$; **** $p < 0.001$.

3. For the *self-drawings*, the massage therapy versus the video control group had lower problem scores on their last day drawings versus their first day drawings. A girl's self-drawing, for example, on the first day was very small, had dark colors and no facial features (see Fig. 4.1a). By the last day, she drew a birthday party with balloons, sunshine and birds, and friends attending the party (Fig. 4.1b).

4. for the *Relaxation Level Rating*, the massage therapy versus the video control children's ratings increased from pre to post on the first day and on the last day, and a significant increase was also noted between baseline ratings on the first day and the last day.

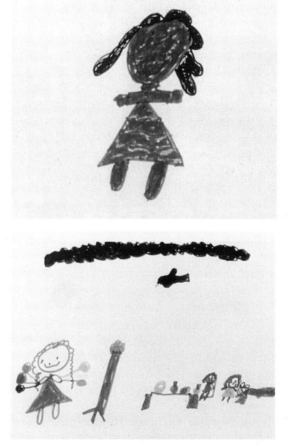

a

b

**Figure 4.1**   Self-drawings by a girl who suffered post-traumatic stress as a result of Hurricane Andrew: (a) drawn before massage therapy study; (b) drawn at end of study

*Discussion*

Like several other post-traumatic stress disorder studies on children, the children exposed to Hurricane Andrew in the area that was most severely hit by the storm experienced severe levels of symptoms, based on Frederick's Post-traumatic Distress Reaction Index. Similarly high Reaction Index scores have been noted following other disasters, including the sniper attack on the elementary school playground in Los Angeles (Pynoos et al 1987), Hurricane Hugo (Lonigan et al 1991), Three Mile Island (Dohrenwend et al 1981), and the Mt St Helena's Volcano (Adams & Adams 1984).

Consistent with some and inconsistent with other studies, there was no apparent relationship between age and sex and the variables tapped in this study, including the scores on the Reaction Index. The data of Lonigan et al (1991) on Hurricane Hugo suggest that girls were more anxious and had a greater number of PTSD symptoms than boys, and black children were more likely than white children to report PTSD symptomatology (Lonigan et al 1991). Similarly, the follow-up study of the children who experienced the Buffalo Creek Dam collapse suggested that there was a greater number of PTSD symptoms in the girls and in the grade school versus preschool age children (Green et al 1991). However, no sex or age differences were noted by Pynoos et al (1987) following the LA sniper attack, nor were sex or age differences noted following the survival of the sinking of the cruise ship Jupiter in Athens harbor in 1988 (Yule 1992).

Some have noted the greater incidence of symptoms in children who experienced greater exposure. For example, the greater-exposure children in the Hurricane Hugo study (Lonigan et al 1991), and the closer-proximity children in the playground sniper gunfire study (Pynoos et al 1987) experienced greater distress. However, we were unable to assess this variable in the present study because of the relatively homogeneous scores on the Hurricane Impact Scale. The homogeneity is perhaps not surprising given that all children were sampled from the grade school located in the middle of the most severely affected area.

In addition to the Hurricane Impact and Reaction Index Scores being in the severe range, the Children's Manifest Anxiety Scale Scores were high for this sample, not unlike other disaster samples such as the Hurricane Hugo sample (Lonigan et al 1991). Similarly, their high depression scale scores (higher than the clinical cutoff for the CESD) are also consistent with other studies such as the study on the sinking of the cruise ship Jupiter (Yule 1992).

Finding a context in the literature for the intervention effects was very disappointing. While the literature search yielded at least a dozen studies on PTSD in children conducted over the last few years, only one intervention study appeared in the literature. In the present study positive effects of the massage therapy were noted immediately after the therapy for all the measures, including the STAI, the Smiley Face Scale, and salivary cortisol levels. These changes were noted only for the massage therapy group on each of the days that the measures were taken: the first day of the study and the last day of the study. In addition, the massage therapy group showed longer-term changes as manifested by lower scores on the Children's Manifest Anxiety Scale, the Center for Epidemiological Studies Depression Scale, and their self-drawings and higher relaxation ratings. Despite the absence of comparison treatment studies in the PTSD literature, the effects noted here are very similar to those noted in a recent study on the effects of massage therapy on children hospitalized for depression and conduct disorder (Field et al 1992). In both studies, anxiety and depression levels were decreased as were stress hormones, including norepinephrine and cortisol. Tactile stimulation with pressure, as in massage therapy, is typically accompanied by these changes.

These findings and the absence of other forms of stimulation during the sessions (i.e. therapists were asked not to verbally stimulate the children, and the children were not likely to become attached to a therapist in one session) suggest that the effects resulted from the massage therapy per se. Additional attention was not a likely explanation since both groups received the same amount of additional attention.

Because most of the PTSD children reported being touched by their mothers and touching their mothers only once weekly as opposed to once daily, and since the school had a 'no touch' policy to reduce potential sexual abuse incidents, these children may have been significantly deprived of physical contact. In that case, it would not be surprising that the children benefitted significantly from the active physical contact of massage therapy. The positive effects at all levels, including self-report scores, drawings, behavioral observation, and biochemical assays are perhaps not surprising, nor are the effects across both anxiety and depression measures given that massage therapy has been noted to have these effects on children – for example, the children hospitalized for psychiatric problems in the study already mentioned (Field et al 1992).

The positive intervention effects are promising given the persistence of PTSD symptoms noted for children who have not received intervention. Those symptoms have persisted for various intervals following disasters such as 1 year after the sinking of the cruise ship Jupiter (Yule 1992), 2 years after the Buffalo Creek Dam collapse disaster (Green et al 1991) and other intervals in the follow-up studies mentioned in the introduction. The question of whether these positive effects persist after termination of the massage therapy must be addressed by a follow-up study. As in many other forms of therapy (nondrug or drug), the treatment effects may not persist following the termination of therapy.

Unlike several other forms of treatment, such as psychotherapy or pharmacological treatment, massage therapy could be continued in a cost-effective way if it were taught to parents, for example, who could massage their children at bedtime on a daily basis. In another application, teachers, even in a school system with a 'no touch' policy, might be given permission to give head/shoulders/ back rubs, and even children's peers could give back rubs as a socially sanctioned form of physical contact. The other advantage of this form of treatment for PTSD children is the ease with which treatment could be immediately administered, for example, by relief workers who would be simultaneously benefitting from administering the massage therapy along with feeling they were helping meet the child's physical as well as psychological needs.

# DEPRESSION IN CHILDREN AND ADOLESCENTS

## Study 2: Massage reduces anxiety in child and adolescent psychiatric patients

Emotional disturbances like depression and adjustment disorder are typically accompanied by anxiety, muscle tension, increased cortisol levels, and sleep disturbances. Anxiety as well as anxious behavior and physiology can be reduced by relaxation therapy (Richter 1984). In one study, relaxation therapy was the most effective treatment (more effective than cognitive behavior therapy) for reducing anxiety in depressed adolescents (Reynolds and Coats 1986). This effect persisted after the end of ten 15-minute sessions. In another study, adolescent psychiatric patients showed less acting-out behavior after relaxation therapy (Corder, Whiteside & Haslip 1986). Finally, in a study on adjustment disorder and depressed child and adolescent patients, both diagnostic groups apeared to benefit from relaxation therapy (Platania-Solazzo et al 1992). Decreases were noted in both self-reported anxiety and in anxious behavior and fidgeting, and increases were observed in positive affect after a 1-hour session of relaxation therapy. Because relaxation therapy is typically composed of several components, including yoga, massage, progressive muscle relaxation, and visual imagery, it is not clear whether any of the individual components, such as massage, can by itself reduce anxiety in these patients.

The present study examined the independent effects of the massage component on the behaviors and physiology of children and adolescents who were hospitalized for depression or adjustment disorder. The massage component was selected because concern has been expressed about touch deprivation in hospitalized children. Depression and adjustment disorder diagnoses were targeted because of their prevalence among hospitalized child and adolescent psychiatric patients. The control group (composed of subjects having either diagnosis) simply viewed a relaxing videotape for the same time as the massage sessions. This group was included to control for the effects of additional care and attention as well as the effects of activity level changes.

## Method

**Sample**  The sample was comprised of 72 children and adolescents (40 boys, 32 girls). Subjects ranged in age from 7 to 18 years (mean = 13). Thirty-six subjects were diagnosed as having adjustment disorder problems (a category that also included conduct disorder and oppositional disorder, conditions that were labeled adjustment disorder for insurance purposes). The remaining 36 subjects were diagnosed as having depression or dysthymic disorder. These diagnoses were made after a 1-hour intake interview by a staff psychiatrist who employed DSM-III-R criteria. Conduct disorder and oppositional defiant disorder were grouped under adjustment disorder, and depression and dysthymia under depressed. These conditions are often comorbid, and we were more interested in assessing the massage effects on externalizing versus internalizing type disorders. The subjects came from lower socioeconomic backgrounds, and the ethnic distribution was approximately 40% Caucasian, 40% Latin, and 20% Black. The subjects were hospitalized for a mean of 21 days (range = 9–64 days).

After group assignment by a random stratification procedure (stratified for sex, age, and medication), comparisons were made between the massage group of 26 adjustment disorder (14 boys), 26 depressed subjects (14 boys), and the control group ($N = 20$: 10 adjustment disorder and 10 depressed) on background factors. No significant differences were noted between the adjustment disorder patients and depressed patients or between the massage and video groups on sex distribution, age, intelligence quotient (mean = 105.7), number of previous admissions (mean = 1.2), duration of hospital stay (mean = 24.6 days), or medications (approximately 30% of each group were receiving medications; the groups were stratified on medications). Several children or adolescents were ineligible for the study because of complex combinations and timing of medications. Because of the increasingly popular notion of comorbidity (on internalizing and externalizing problems), antidepressants were the most commonly used medication on our adolescent units. Thirty percent of the adjustment disorder and 30% of the depressed groups were receiving antidepressants, and none of the children or adolescents had received that medication longer than a week at the time of their entry into the study. Thus, it was hoped, the medication did not differentially influence the behaviors or the biochemical levels (cortisol and catecholamines) of the groups.

**Massage**   The massage group subjects received 30 minutes of moderate pressure back massage per day for 5 days. The massage consisted of carefully timed stroking movements for 5-minute periods in each of three regions: up and down the neck, from the neck across the shoulders and back to the neck, and from the neck to the waist and back to the neck along the vertebral column. The 15-minute sequence was comprised of 30 back-and-forth strokes per region at 10 seconds each. This same 15-minute sequence was repeated in its entirety for a total of a 30 minutes massage. The massages were given at the same time of day (midafternoon) over the 5-day period, and they were administered by psychology students trained in the standard massage procedure. Male psychology students administered massage to male patients and female students to female patients The subjects were told that it was hoped that the procedure (both massage and relaxing video-tape) would help them relax. After the procedure, the subjects were asked if they liked the treatment and if it made them feel relaxed. The relaxing nature of the massage and video conditions was evident by the subjects' self-reports after the sessions. Although this is a subjective measure, the reduction in activity level in both conditions is also suggestive of the relaxing nature of the conditions. The psychology students were instructed not to talk during the massage (and video conditions) except to ask the subjects after the massage (and video conditions) if they liked the treatment and if it made them feel relaxed. The psychology students were asked not to talk for two reasons: (1) a massage without talking is generally considered more relaxing; (2) during the piloting, massage often facilitated self-disclosure in the subjects. Because the psychology students were not the subjects' primary therapists, self-disclosure was not encouraged during these sessions. The nurses were 'blind' to the condition (massage or video) of the patients (although certainly not to the diagnosis) because the patients were seen in a closed room for similar periods of time and were requested not to reveal their condition. 'Keeping a secret from staff' was something that appealed to these youngsters, and by the nurses' report, they did not know the subjects' condition.

**Videotape viewing control condition** The control group was seen at the same time of day for a videotape viewing session for the same period of time (30 minutes per day for 5 days). During this condition, the patient simply sat and watched a relaxing video-tape (of pleasant sounds and visual images) with the student. The patient was asked to remain still and quiet for the 30-minute sessions. This control condition was employed to ensure that any changes noted in behavior or physiology during the massage sessions were not simply related to temporal or activity variation in these measures, to clinical improvement from other treatments, or from the physical presence and attention provided by the student. The same measurements as those used in the massage condition were employed in the control condition over the same time frame for the subsample of 20 subjects.

**Assessments** The assessments included self-reports of anxiety and depression, behavioral observations, nurse ratings of the same behaviors that were included in the behavioral observation schedule, actometer readings of activity level, heart rate, saliva samples for cortisol, urine samples for cortisol and catecholamines (norepinephrine, epinephrine, and dopamine), and time-lapse videotaping of night-time sleep sessions. On the first and last days of the treatment period, baseline, presession, postsession, and follow-up assessment measures were collected according to the following schedule:

1. 30 minutes before the massage and/or video session (baseline): the State Anxiety Scale for Children (Spielberger et al 1973)
2. immediately before the massage and/or video session: saliva samples, activity level, pulse rate, and behavior observation ratings based on the previous 30 minutes of the subjects' baseline behavior
3. immediately after the massage and/or video session: activity level, pulse rate, behavior ratings based on behavior noted during the session, and self-report measures
4. 30 minutes after the massage and/or video session (follow-up): saliva samples, activity level, pulse rate, and behavior ratings based on the previous 30 minutes of postsession behavior.

The three different time periods are referred to in the tables as pre, post, and 30 minute post periods. Finally, on the first and last treatment days, night-time sleep was videotaped using a time-lapse video camera, and subjects were asked to collect a 24-hour urine sample to be assayed for urine cortisol and catecholamines (norepinephrine, epinephrine, and dopamine). To ensure subject compliance, the children and adolescents were given a game or audiotape of their choice after the 5-day period.

*Self-report measures.* The *self-report measures* taken before and after the first and last sessions included: *The STAIC* (Spielberger et al 1973) and *The Profile of Mood States* (POMS) (McNair et al 1971).

*Behavior observation ratings.* Behavior observation ratings were completed three times based on behavior observed as follows: (a) during the 30 minutes before the sessions (data are given under 'pre' in the tables); (b) during the sessions themselves (post); (c) during the 30-minute period after the sessions were completed (follow-up). For a more objective measure of the subjects' *activity level*, an actometer was used. The actometer is a Timex watch that has been adapted to cumulatively record movements in the horizontal and vertical plane. It is worn on the subject's wrist like a typical watch. Activity level was calculated by subtracting the reading taken from the monitor at the beginning from the reading taken at the end of each observation period (pre, during, and post the massage). The difference was then divided by the number of seconds that had elapsed and multiplied by 100 to yield a whole number.

*Other measures.* *Pulse rate* was measured by taking the subject's radial pulse for 30 seconds before, after, and 30 minutes after the end of each session. *Saliva cortisol samples* were collected at the same times (Appendix 2A).

Twenty-four hour *urine samples* were collected by the subjects (approximately evenly distributed across groups) under the supervision of the nursing staff. An aliquot of each 24-hour sample was frozen and sent to Duke University for subsequent assays. Urinary levels of norepinephrine and epinephrine were analyzed by high-pressure liquid chromatography with electrochemical detection.

*Night-time sleep recordings.* Night-time sleep was videotaped on the first and last treatment days using a time-lapse videocamera. The videocamera was set up on a tripod in the subject's room to focus on the bed of the subject. The subject (under the supervision of the nursing staff) was responsible for turning the camera on at bedtime and turning it off next morning. The videotapes were subsequently coded using a time-lapse video system enabling

8 hours of videotape to be coded in 2 hours. The tapes were coded for quiet sleep (no body movement), active sleep (body movement), awake and lying quietly, and awake and active.

## Results

Tables 4.3 and 4.4 feature the mean values for the measures pre, post, and 30 minutes after (follow-up) the massage and video sessions on the first day (Day 1) and the last day (Day 5) of the massage treatment period. The average values for the diagnostic groups are given here because there were no diagnostic group differences.

**Immediate effects of massage** As can be seen in Table 4.3, the following immediate effects of massage were noted.

1. For the self-report measures: a significant decrease in STAIC scores was recorded between the pre and follow-up measures on both Days 1 and 5, and, for the POMS Scale, the score decreased from pre to follow-up on Day 1 but not on Day 5.

2. Based on the behavior observations, the following changes occurred: the state ratings decreased during the massage, suggesting that the patients were less alert during the massage; the affect ratings increased and remained elevated at follow-up, indicating that the patients were showing more positive affect after the massage; the vocalization ratings decreased during the massage and returned to baseline following the sessions; activity level decreased during both the massage and the video sessions and returned to baseline at the end of the sessions; and, anxiety and fidgeting ratings decreased during the massage and remained diminished at follow-up, suggesting that the patients were showing less anxiety and fidgeting behavior during and after the massage.

3. Like the behavior observation ratings on activity, the actometer readings on Day 1 decreased during the massage and video sessions and remained low, although on Day 5 the readings decreased but then returned to baseline.

4. Similarly, pulse decreased and remained decreased during the massage and video sessions on Day 1 and decreased but returned to baseline on Day 5.

5. Saliva cortisol levels decreased, but only during massage, and remained diminished at the 30-minute follow-up period.

**Longer-term effects of massage** Several effects were noted for the Day 1 and Day 5 values, suggesting changes for the massage group, although no changes occurred for the video group. The changes for the massage group were as follows (Table 4.3).

**Table 4.3**  Mean values[1] for self-report and behavior measures pre, post, and 30 minutes after massage on first day (Day 1) and last day (Day 5) of massage treatment period (Study 2)

| Measures | First day (Day 1) | | | Last day (Day 5) | | |
|---|---|---|---|---|---|---|
| | Pre | Post | 30 min post | Pre | Post | 30 min post |
| Self-report | | | | | | |
| State Anxiety | 34.7 | 27.3 | 31.9 | 27.6 | | |
| | 33.8 | 31.9 | 31.8 | 29.3 | | |
| POMS | 20.4 | 16.4 | 14.7 | 14.7 | | |
| | 16.3 | 14.5 | 13.5 | 13.0 | | |
| Behavior observation ratings | | | | | | |
| State | 2.4 | 1.5****[2] | 2.6 | 2.5 | 1.7**** | 2.6 |
| | 2.7 | 2.5 | 2.7 | 2.8 | 2.7 | 2.8 |
| Affect | 2.0 | 2.3*** | 2.3*** | 2.0 | 2.3** | 2.2* |
| | 2.2 | 2.1 | 2.2 | 2.3 | 2.4 | 2.5 |
| Vocalizations | 1.8 | 1.1*** | 1.8 | 1.8 | 1.2**** | 1.9 |
| | 1.8 | 1.6 | 1.9 | 1.8 | 1.8 | 1.8 |
| Activity | 1.7 | 1.2**** | 1.8 | 1.7 | 1.4**** | 1.8 |
| | 1.7 | 1.3*** | 1.7 | 2.0 | 1.5*** | 1.8 |
| Anxiety | 1.7 | 1.2 | 1.3*** | 1.4* | 1.2* | 1.2* |
| | 1.5 | 1.6 | 1.4 | 1.6 | 1.5 | 1.6 |
| Fidgeting | 1.5 | 1.2** | 1.2** | 1.4 | 1.1* | 1.2* |
| | 1.3 | 1.3 | 1.3 | 1.3 | 1.3 | 1.3 |
| Cooperation | 2.8 | 2.9 | 2.8 | 2.8 | 2.8 | 2.8 |
| | 2.8 | 2.9 | 2.9 | 2.9 | 2.9 | 2.8 |
| Nurses' ratings | | | | | | |
| State | 2.8 | | | 2.9 | | |
| | 2.9 | | | 2.9 | | |
| Affect | 1.9 | | | 2.3* | | |
| | 1.9 | | | 2.0 | | |
| Vocalizations | 2.1 | | | 2.2 | | |
| | 2.4 | | | 2.4 | | |
| Activity | 2.3 | | | 2.5 | | |
| | 2.6 | | | 2.6 | | |
| Anxiety | 2.1 | | | 1.8* | | |
| | 2.0 | | | 1.9 | | |
| Fidgeting | 1.8 | | | 1.5* | | |
| | 1.6 | | | 1.6 | | |
| Cooperation | 2.1 | | | 2.3* | | |
| | 2.2 | | | 2.3 | | |

[1] Video group means appear below massage group means in each pair of rows.
[2] Asterisks after post means are pre–post session comparisons. Asterisks after pre means last day (Day 5) are for comparisons between Day 1 and Day 5 baseline (pre) means: * $p = 0.05$, ** $p = 0.01$, *** $p = 0.005$, **** $p = 0.001$.

1.   For the self-report measures: the STAIC score was lower at baseline on Day 5 than it was on Day 1, but only for the depressed group. The mean score for the depressed group decreased from 37 to 33, whereas a negligible change was noted in the adjustment disorder group. For the POMS scale, however, the scores of both of the diagnostic groups decreased, indicating a less depressed mood by Day 5.

**Table 4.4** Mean values[1] for physiological and sleep measures pre, post, and 30 minutes after massage on first day (Day 1) and last day (Day 5) of massage treatment period (Study 2)

| Measures | First day (Day 1) | | | Last day (Day 5) | | |
|---|---|---|---|---|---|---|
| | Pre | Post | 30 min post | Pre | Post | 30 min post |
| **Physiological measures** | | | | | | |
| Activity watch | 5.0 | 1.5****[2] | 3.6* | 3.4* | 1.7** | 3.6 |
| | 3.8 | 2.6** | 3.1 | 3.8 | 2.4** | 3.1 |
| Pulse | 88.0 | 79.0**** | 82.0*** | 87.0 | 82.0**** | 85.0 |
| | 86.0 | 80.0** | 84.0 | 84.0 | 80.0 | 87.0 |
| Saliva cortisol | 1.8 | 1.4* | 1.3** | 2.2 | 1.4**** | 1.6**** |
| | 1.7 | 1.7 | 1.9 | 1.9 | 1.7 | 1.6 |
| Urine cortisol | 87.4 | | | 78.7** | | |
| | 82.7 | | | 86.1 | | |
| Norepinephrine | 29.6 | | | 25.2 | | |
| | 27.6 | | | 29.5 | | |
| Epinephrine | 4.3 | | | 4.0 | | |
| | 4.4 | | | 4.7 | | |
| Dopamine | 265.0 | | | 261.0 | | |
| | 271.8 | | | 286.7 | | |
| **Sleep behaviors** | | | | | | |
| Time asleep | 79.7 | | | 91.3** | | |
| | 82.1 | | | 84.5 | | |
| **States 1 & 2** | | | | | | |
| Time awake (%) | 15.2 | | | 4.0* | | |
| | 15.6 | | | 17.9 | | |

[1] Video group means appear below massage group means in each pair of rows.
[2] Asterisks after post means are pre–post session comparisons. Asterisks after pre means last day (Day 5) are for comparisons between Day 1 and Day 5 baseline (pre) means:
* $p = 0.05$; ** $p = 0.01$; *** $p = 0.005$; **** $p = 0.001$.

2. Based on the behavior observations: both diagnostic groups that were massaged showed a decrease in anxiety-like behavior from Day 1 to Day 5; the depressed group versus the adjustment disorder group had lower activity levels (based on behavior observation and activity watch) and fidgeting behavior on Day 5.

3. Based on the nurses' ratings of behavior on the unit, positive changes were noted to occur over the 5-day period, including an increase in positive affect, a decrease in anxiety and fidgeting behavior, and an increase in cooperative behavior.

4. Saliva cortisol levels did not change over the 5-day period, although the depressed group had lower saliva cortisol levels than the adjustment disorder group on Day 5.

5. Urine cortisol significantly decreased over the 5-day period, but this decrease occurred only for the depressed group (for depressed group, Day 1 cortisol mean = 99, Day 5 = 64, and for the adjustment disorder group Day 1 cortisol mean = 80, Day 5 = 85).

6. Similarly, urine norepinephrine decreased, but only for the depressed group (for the depressed group, Day 1 norepinephrine mean = 39, Day 5 = 29, and for the adjustment disorder group, Day 1 mean = 27, Day 5 = 25).

7. Based on the time-lapse video of the night-time sleep sessions, the percentage of time in bed for which sleep occurred increased over the 5-day period, and the percentage of time for which night-time wakefulness occurred correspondingly decreased over the same period for the massage group.

## Discussion

After the massage sessions, patients' self-reported anxiety scores (STAIC) and depression scores (POMS) decreased significantly. Likewise, ratings on the Behavior Observation Scale also improved immediately after the massage sessions. The children and adolescents showed more positive affect and less anxiety and fidgeting behavior. In addition, although decreases were noted in activity level and heart rate during both the massage and video sessions, decreases in saliva cortisol levels only occurred during the massage sessions. This finding from the control video group suggests that the decrease noted in saliva cortisol levels during massage was probably unrelated to decreased activity level. The consistency of these results across diagnostic groups and the convergence of self-report, behavioral, physiological and biochemical measures in the direction of less anxiety highlights the immediate effectiveness of the massage treatment. Additional evidence for the specific effectiveness of massage is provided by the comparison with the video control group, who merely showed diminished activity level and heart rate during the sessions. The longer-term effects of the massage treatment across the 5-day period were probably of greater

**Table 4.5** Mean values for measures on which the depressed and adjustment disorder children and adolescents of the massage group differed (Study 2)

| | Means | | | |
| --- | --- | --- | --- | --- |
| | Depressed | | Adjustment disorder | |
| | Day 1 | Day 5 | Day 1 | Day 5 |
| State anxiety | 37 | 33* | 32 | 31 |
| Urine cortisol | 99 | 64** | 80 | 85 |
| Urine norepinephrine | 39 | 29* | 27 | 25 |

* $p < 0.05$; ** $p < 0.001$.

clinical importance. Although no long-term changes were noted in the video group, significant changes occurred in the massage group. Self-reported depression levels were lower by the end of the 5-day period for both diagnostic groups that were massaged, and lower state anxiety scores were noted in the depressed massage group. Even though the adjustment disorder group anxiety levels did not change according to self report, behavior observations and nurses' ratings of anxiety suggested that both groups were lower on anxiety. The nurses also rated fidgeting behavior as occurring less often, and they noted improved affect and cooperation by the last day of treatment. In addition, by the end of the 5-day period, the children and adolescents were spending more of their bedtime periods in sleep and less time awake. Finally, the depressed group showed some changes not evident in the adjustment disorder group, including decreases in urine cortisol and norepinephrine levels.

The consistency of this self-report and behavior observation data, and the positive immediate and longer-term effects of the massage treatment, support the use of this treatment for children and adolescents on psychiatric units. Although the immediate effects of the massage were anticipated, we had not expected the positive effects to persist across the treatment period. Of particular clinical importance were the nurses' ratings of the children as being more cooperative and less depressed, anxious, and fidgeting. Thus, it would appear that the effects were not limited to the massage treatment period but generalized to behavior on the unit, as observed by the nurses.

The longer-term effects were more pronounced for the depressed versus the adjustment disorder children and adolescents (Table 4.5). Although anxious behavior, based on observer and nurse behavior ratings, decreased in the adjustment disorder children over the 5-day period, their self-reported anxiety levels started at lower levels than the depressed patients and remained the same over the massage period. Their cortisol and norepinephrine levels were similarly lower and did not change over the 5-day period. Although the massage appeared, then, to reduce behavioral anxiety in these children, they apparently were less affected by the massage treatments at a feeling and biochemical level. As in an initial level effect, it is not surprising that a high baseline level of physiological or biochemical activity might diminish with treatment, whereas low baseline levels would remain the same. It is also possible that while the adjustment disorder children showed immediate effects of the massage, they were unaffected by the treatment over the long-term and simply displayed the expected and desirable reduction in anxious behavior immediately after the sessions. Alternatively, depressed children may simply be more sensitive or responsive to physical stimulation of this kind.

Several limitations of these findings can be noted. Certainly, longer-term follow-up data would be desirably collected on another sample for both replication and follow-up purposes. With respect to potential abuses of massage, some concerns were raised by clinicians on these psychiatric units. One was the concern that staff may be accused of sexual abuse for extensive touching of patients (during the massage). For this reason, the massage was limited to the head and back regions, and the patients were fully clothed. Because of the same concern, therapists who were the same sex as the patients gave the massage. A potentially more desirable arrangement is the use of grandmother or grandfather volunteer massage therapists to attenuate this problem as well as to reduce treatment costs. The use of same-sex therapists raised the potential concern about patients with homosexual tendencies or history of sex abuse. For this problem, the psychiatric staff advised that cues (verbal or nonverbal) be taken from the individual patient who might or might not experience massage as an aversive treatment.

Although the clinical staff in general supported the use of massage in these patients' treatment, particularly in light of their concern about the infrequency of touching received by these children during their hospitalization, they were also concerned about how their children would react to extensive touch, i.e., the massage. Many of the children did not recall ever having been touched by their parents, and none of the children had ever received a massage. In addition, the staff were concerned that massage would be popularized on the unit, leading to adolescent-to-adolescent massage and potential promiscuity. This problem did not occur, at least during the course of the study.

Finally, the staff was concerned about the facilitating effects of massage on self-disclosure of intimate material by the patients. Although pilot data suggested that massage could be effectively used for this reason by primary therapists, the massage therapists in this research were not primary therapists. Simply instructing the massage therapists to behave like 'real masseurs,' who do not talk, effectively discouraged self-disclosure. After resolving these problems anticipated by the staff, the only remaining problem expressed by the staff was that they, too, needed massage to reduce their stress.

On a different note, the parameters of the massage used were somewhat arbitrary. Midafternoon was selected because the adolescents tended to be more aroused at that time, probably because it marked the end of their school period. A period of 30 minutes was chosen because it is the typical duration for commercial massages in hotels and sports clubs. Variables such as these and the use of primary therapists and same sex therapists for massage treatment will require further investigation.

These data do not clarify whether the treatment effects noted in relaxation therapy studies (Platania-Solazzo et al 1992, Reynolds and Coats 1986, Richter 1984) derived from massage per se, or from other relaxation therapy components, such as progressive muscle relaxation, exercise, or yoga. Nonetheless, the data from the self-reports, behavioral observations, and cortisol levels converged to suggest reduced anxiety over the short term as well as decreases in anxiety over the long term for at least the depressed subjects. Moreover, the nursing staff's ratings concurred with the behavioral observation ratings, suggesting that massage may have positive effects on hospitalized child and adolescent psychiatric patients with either depression or adjustment disorder. In another study (reported next) depressed adolescent mothers who received massage therapy experienced very similar effects.

## Study 3: Massage and relaxation therapies' effects on depressed adolescent mothers

Depression is one of the most prevalent medical disorders and has been recognized as a distinct pathologic entity from early Egyptian times. Anxiety is one of the primary features of depression in adolescents. Relaxation therapy (RT) is usually noted to decrease anxiety. Using the STAI, for example, anxiety levels were lower in psychiatric patients following nine sessions of relaxation therapy (Hosmand et al 1985). Even following one brief RT session, mood was elevated on the Profile of Mood States Scale (Matthew & Gelder, 1969).

In a longer-term outcome study RT was as effective as psychotherapy and pharmacotherapy in reducing anxiety (McLean & Hakistian 1979) and even more effective than cognitive behavior therapy (Reynolds & Coats 1986). Similarly, in a study on depressed child and adolescent psychiatric patients, both groups benefitted from as little as one hour of relaxation therapy (Platania-Solazzo et al 1992). Self-reported anxiety as well as anxious behavior and fidgeting decreased, and increases were noted in positive affect.

Massage therapy (MT), with child and adolescent psychiatric patients led to lower anxiety levels, more optimal affect and sleep patterns, and lower stress hormones in the study just reviewed (Field et al 1992) and was therefore expected to have similar effects on depressed adolescent mothers. Massage and relaxation therapy may be even more important for depressed adolescents who are mothers. Maternal depression ranges from 25–30% during the first 3 months after delivery (O'Hara, Neunaber & Zekoski 1984). Even mild depression and anxiety may affect the new mother's relationship with her child. For example, in one study, postpartum depressed mothers showed less rocking, gaze, and positive regard toward their infants than nondepressed mothers (Livingood, Dean & Smith 1983). Others have reported less-frequent positive states and more-frequent negative states among depressed mother–infant dyads (Cohn et al 1990, Field et al 1990). Thus, methods are needed for reducing anxiety and depression in the mothers.

## Method

**Sample** The sample was comprised of 32 depressed adolescent mothers who had recently given birth at a large inner city hospital and were recruited from the hospital's maternity ward. The subjects were randomly assigned to the massage therapy or relaxation therapy group. The groups did not differ on age (mean = 18.1), years of education (mean = 10.4), ethnicity (71% Black, 29% Hispanic), or SES (mean = 4.7 on the Hollingshead Index). To qualify for the study the mothers needed to have an elevated Beck Depression Inventory (BDI) score and needed to be free of current medication or other treatment for depression or related disorders. The depression classification was based on a diagnosis of dysthymia on the Diagnostic Inventory Schedule (Costello, Edelbrock & Costello 1985) and a score greater than 16 on the Beck Depression Inventory (Beck et al 1961).

### Treatment procedures

*Massage therapy.* The massage therapy subjects ($N = 16$) received a 30-minute massage per day on 2 consecutive days per week for 5 consecutive weeks (10 massages). For the first 15 minutes the subject was in a supine position for massage in the following four regions:

1. head/neck – slow lateral stroking of forehead, followed by long and slow stroking from the neck across the shoulders and from the shoulders to the neck
2. arms/hands – long and slow stroking from above the shoulder to beyond the hand, followed by individual stroking of each hand

3. torso – placing the hand gently on the solar plexus (base of chest) and adding a gentle rocking motion
4. legs/feet – long, slow stroking from the hip to beyond the foot, followed by stroking each foot.

For the second 15 minutes the subject was in a prone position. This segment consisted of an achilles tendon (ankle) stretch (bend the knee to stretch), knee and calf shake, long and slow strokes from over the buttocks to the toes, lateral lumbar stretch (10 times) including strokes parallel to the spine from the base of the spine to the shoulders and along the arms to past the end of the hands, trapezius (shoulder blade) squeeze, friction alongside the spine with the ulnar (outside) edge of the hand from superior to inferior, posterior neck squeeze and stretch, and long slow strokes from the head down the entire posterior surface of the body to the toes (three times). The massage therapy was administered by trained massage therapists and performed at the same time of day (mid-afternoon) over the 5-week period.

*Relaxation therapy.* The relaxation therapy subjects (N = 16) spent the same amount of time in RT as the massage therapy subjects spent in MT. They attended 30-minute relaxation therapy sessions on two consecutive days a week for five consecutive weeks (10 sessions). The subjects used exercise mats, and the first 15 minutes of the session consisted of yoga exercises. The second 15-minute segment consisted of progressive muscle relaxation. For this relaxation, the subjects were instructed to breathe deeply for several minutes, and the instructor asked the subjects to relax and tense eight different muscle groups, beginning with the feet and ending with the head. The same measures as those used in the massage/ control conditions were used in the relaxation therapy condition over the same time frame.

**Assessment procedures** The effects of the massage and relaxation therapies were assessed as follows on the first and last days of the assessment period: (a) *Behavior Observation Scales* (Platania-Solazzo et al 1992); (b) *Profile of Mood States* (POMS) (McNair et al 1971); (c) *STAIC* (Spielberger et al 1973); (d) *pulse rate*; (e) *saliva samples of cortisol* (Appendix 2A); (f) *urine sample for cortisol*. On the first and last days of the treatment period the baseline, during session, and postsession assessment measures were collected according to the following schedule: (1) *30 minutes prior to the treatment condition*: STAIC and POMS; (2) *immediately prior to the treatment condition*: pulse rate, saliva samples, and behavior observation ratings based on the previous 30 minutes of the subjects' behavior; (3) *immediately after the session*: pulse rate, STAIC, POMS, behavior ratings based on the previous 30 minutes of behavior, saliva and urine samples were taken; (4) *30 minutes after the session*: because of the 20-minute lag time, saliva samples were taken for cortisol assays 30 minutes after the session to tap the cortisol levels at the end of the session. These samples were frozen and sent to Dr Saul Schanberg's laboratory at Duke University for analysis.

## Results

The groups were comparable on demographic variables, including maternal age, SES, ethnicity, and initial BDI score.

The data analyses suggested the following (Tables 4.6, 4.7).

1. State anxiety decreased for the massage therapy group following the first and last day therapy sessions and only on the first day for the relaxation group.

2. POMS depression scores were lower following the massage on the first and last days.

3. Behavior Observation Scale ratings favored the massage therapy group, including:
(a) a higher state rating after therapy on day 10
(b) higher vocalization ratings after therapy on days 1 and 10
(c) lower anxiety ratings after the massage therapy sessions on days 1 and 10
(d) higher cooperation ratings for the MT group after therapy on days 1 and 10
(e) fidgetiness decreased for the MT group on both the first and last days.

4. Pulse rate decreased after massage therapy on days 1 and 10.

5. Salivary cortisol levels were lower after massage therapy.

6. Urine cortisol levels were lower on the last day than on the first day of massage therapy.

## Discussion

The relaxation group reported lower anxiety levels on the first day, but only the massage therapy group reported less anxiety *and* showed less anxious behavior and lower stress hormone (cortisol) levels after their sessions. In addition, only the massage therapy group experienced a reduction in depression and in stress (as manifested by their lower urinary cortisol levels) across the course of the study. These results are consistent with several studies in the literature using self-reports to tap anxiety levels following relaxation therapy (McLean & Hakistian 1979, Platania-

**Table 4.6**    Means for massage therapy group (Study 3)

|  | Day 1 | | Day 10 | |
| --- | --- | --- | --- | --- |
|  | Pre | Post | Pre | Post |
| State Anxiety Scale | 35.67**** | 28.67 | 33.89*** | 28.28 |
| POMS Depression | 19.44* | 11.43 | 20.39*** | 9.06 |
| Behavior Observation Scale |  |  |  |  |
| State | 2.22 | 2.29 | 2.09 | 2.11 |
| Affect | 1.72***** | 2.67 | 1.67**** | 2.83 |
| Activity | 1.61 | 1.67 | 1.69 | 1.50 |
| Vocalization | 1.44* | 1.83 | 1.50** | 1.94 |
| Anxiety | 1.83**** | 1.06 | 1.94**** | 1.06 |
| Cooperation | 2.50**** | 2.89 | 2.17**** | 2.89 |
| Fidgetiness | 1.61** | 1.11 | 1.61*** | 1.11 |
| Pulse | 85.06**** | 77.76 | 87.88**** | 77.65 |
| Saliva cortisol | 1.21** | 0.84 | 1.55* | 1.16 |
| Urine cortisol | 166.95* |  | 120.08 |  |

Asterisks indicate significant differences between adjacent means: $* p < 0.05$; $** p < 0.01$; $*** p < 0.005$; $**** p < 0.001$.

**Table 4.7**    Means for relaxation therapy group (Study 3)

|  | Day 1 | | Day 10 | |
| --- | --- | --- | --- | --- |
|  | Pre | Post | Pre | Post |
| State Anxiety Scale | 34.73* | 31.55 | 33.09 | 31.73 |
| POMS Depression | 18.37 | 19.40 | 18.56 | 17.12 |
| Behavior Observation Scale |  |  |  |  |
| State | 2.20 | 2.10 | 2.45 | 2.00 |
| Affect | 2.55 | 2.45 | 2.64 | 2.55 |
| Activity | 1.82 | 1.82 | 1.91 | 1.73 |
| Vocalization | 1.82 | 1.64 | 2.09 | 1.86 |
| Anxiety | 1.55 | 1.55 | 1.18 | 1.09 |
| Cooperation | 2.82 | 2.55 | 2.55 | 2.64 |
| Fidgetiness | 1.36 | 1.00 | 1.09 | 1.00 |
| Pulse | 84.00 | 85.56 | 73.78 | 75.78 |
| Saliva cortisol | 1.55 | 1.65 | 1.87 | 1.30 |
| Urine cortisol | 165.50 |  | 168.39 |  |

Asterisk indicates significant differences between adjacent means: $* p < 0.05$.

Solazzo et al 1992, Reynolds & Coats 1986). The massage therapy data are consistent with the previously described study showing not only a reduction in anxiety and depression by self-report but also by behavior observation and cortisol levels (Field et al 1992). Possible explanations for the differential effects are that a reduction in self-reported anxiety may be a simple placebo effect or the subjects may have felt less anxious after a therapy designed to make them relax but did not show the same effects in their behavior or stress hormones, because they had to work during the relaxation therapy.

Anecdotal reports from the adolescent mothers were that they did not enjoy the relaxation therapy because they had to 'work too hard'. This may explain why they had lower state and cooperation ratings.

The long-term effect of massage therapy on urinary cortisol but not on self-report or observed behavior might relate to urinary cortisol reflecting a cumulative effect of the massage therapy that cannot be controlled by the subjects. In contrast, the behavior and self-report could be controlled by the subjects and may have reflected their current state at the time of the assessment. Many of the subjects expressed disappointment at the end of the study about the massage therapy ending. This might explain their behavior and self-report not showing the cumulative benefit that the urinary cortisol levels did.

Future research might assess relaxation and massage therapy devotees to avoid the bias against 'relaxation therapy as work'. A more passive form of relaxation therapy could also be used as a comparison. In addition, measures could be taken at the penultimate session to avoid the disappointment bias of the last session. The use of convergent self-report, behavioral, physiological, and biochemical measures led to different conclusions than the literature would suggest. But additional research would be needed before concluding that massage therapy has more positive and more long-lasting effects than relaxation therapy for reducing depression and anxiety in depressed adolescent mothers.

## ANOREXIA AND BULIMIA IN WOMEN

Another group of people who experience severe depression are adolescents with eating disorders, including anorexia (undereating) and bulimia (overeating and vomiting).

### Study 4: Bulimic adolescents benefit from massage therapy

Bulimia nervosa was originally thought to be a derivative of anorexia, but it is now recognized as a disorder of its own. A diagnosis of bulimia requires the following symptoms: (a) recurrent episodes of binge eating; (b) a feeling of lack of control over eating behavior during the eating binges; (c) regularly engaging in either self-induced vomiting, use of laxatives or diuretics, strict dieting or fasting, or vigorous exercise in order to prevent weight gain; (d) a minimum average of two binge eating episodes a week for at least 3 months; and (e) persistent overconcern with body shape/weight (American Psychiatric Association 1987).

The exact etiology of bulimia nervosa is not yet determined, but the behaviors and symptoms presented by the majority of patients suggest a combination of psychological, social, and physiological factors. Depressed affect is so commonly seen in bulimics that some believe it is simply a type of affective disorder. 20–30% of patients with bulimia meet the diagnostic criteria for depression (Edelstein, Haskew & Kramer 1989). Bulimic patients who vomit show lower urinary serotonin (Kaye, Ebert & Gwirtsman 1984) but elevated plasma norepinephrine (Robinson, Checkley & Russell 1985, Smythe, Bradshaw & Vining 1983).

Some bulimics are difficult to medicate because those who binge do not keep the medication in their systems long enough to absorb it, some bulimic patients who are not depressed respond to antidepressant medication and some who are depressed may binge less while remaining depressed (Brotman, Herzog & Woods 1984, Walsh et al 1984). Some of the relief experienced by bulimic patients may be due to the lowered anxiety and suppressed appetite caused by tricyclic antidepressants rather than the antidepressant activity itself (Pope & Hudson 1986). Significant decreases in bulimic or depressive symptoms have been demonstrated for tricyclic antidepressants, serotonergic agents, and MAO inhibitors.

None of these treatment approaches has been sufficient on its own. To be successful, treatment must alleviate depressive symptoms and alter any neuro-endocrinological abnormalities. Massage therapy has proven effective in all of these areas, reducing depression and cortisol (Field et al 1992). In our study with depressed adolescents, for example, massage lowered both self-reported and observed anxiety and depression levels as well as salivary cortisol levels.

Given the positive effects noted in depressed adolescents, we expected that massage therapy would be similarly effective with eating disorder patients. We expected decreased depression, anxiety, and cortisol levels. In addition, massage therapy was expected to positively affect the patients' body image. As another form of direct feedback, massage therapy was expected to increase the patients' awareness of their bodies, which is thought to be critical for resolving body perception dissonance (Vandereycken & Meermann 1984). Psychotherapy and pharmacotherapy have been somewhat effective, although the majority of patients have continuing eating problems (Garfinkel, Moldofsky & Garner 1977, Hsu 1986). Massage therapy may be an effective adjunct to these therapies and reduce recidivism.

## Method

**Sample** The subjects were 24 adolescent female bulimic in-patients treated at a residential center. The entry criterion was a

DSM-III-R diagnosis of bulimia nervosa: weight loss is usually present, amenorrhea is variable, vomiting/purging is normally present, as is fear of fatness (Hsu 1986). The patients ranged in age from 16 to 21 and came from middle to upper SES (M = 2.2 on the Hollingshead Index) Hispanic (68%) and Non-Hispanic White (32%) families. The patients were randomly assigned to a massage therapy or a standard treatment control group.

### Treatment procedures

*Massage therapy.* The massage therapy group subjects received a massage twice a week for 5 weeks, for a total of 10 massages. The massages were administered by massage therapists. The massage therapy covered several parts of the body (which was fully clothed) and included 15 minutes in a supine position and 15 minutes in a prone position. It consisted of first exerting traction upon the neck with the patient in a supine position, followed by smooth strokes across the forehead, jaw and face, and depressing the shoulders. The therapist then moved each arm one at a time and exerted traction, followed by massage of the hand and smooth strokes over the length of the arm. The torso was gently rocked, and then the same movements used with the arms were used with the legs and feet, one at a time. In a prone position the Achilles tendon was stretched and long strokes were made from the hip to the toes. The strokes on the back included lateral lumbar stretching, strokes that connect the back and arms, trapezius and neck squeezing, friction alongside the spine, sacral traction and long, soothing strokes from the head to the feet.

*Standard treatment.* All adolescents residing at an eating disorder treatment center were evaluated by a psychiatrist prior to admission to assess their goals and identify a treatment plan. The adolescents then met their primary clinician and participated in daily small groups, individual, family and community therapy sessions. In addition, they worked with a registered dietician to become more knowledgeable about nutritional choices and the basic principles of physiology and metabolism, and they participated in nonverbal therapies such as movement therapy. In total, residents attended 30 to 40 group therapy sessions per week.

### Assessment procedures

*Immediate-effects measures (pre/post therapy sessions).* The immediate effects measures included: (1) the *STAI* (Spielberger et al 1970); (2) The *Profile of Mood States Depression Scale* (POMS–D) (McNair et al 1971); (3) *Behavior Observation Ratings* (Field et al 1992); (4) *saliva cortisol* samples (Appendix 2A).

*Longer-term effects measures (first day/last day).* The longer-term measures included: (1) *Eating Disorders Inventory* (EDI) (Garner,

Olmsted and Polivy 1983); (2) *The Center for Epidemiological Studies Depression Scale* (CES–D) (Radloff 1977); ratings of depression (Radloff & Locke 1986, Radloff 1991); (3) *urine samples* collected from the subjects prior to the end of the first and last day therapy sessions. An aliquot of each sample was frozen and sent to Duke University to be assayed for cortisol, serotonin (5HIAA), creatinine, and catecholamines (norepinephrine, epinephrine, and dopamine). Assays were performed as previously described (Kuhn et al 1991). Serotonin is depleted in bulimics (Kaye et al 1984) and they are noted to have elevated norepinephrine levels (Robinson et al 1985, Smythe, Bradshaw & Vining 1983). In our previous studies massage therapy reduced norepinephrine levels in depressed adolescents and increased serotonin levels in stressed men (Ironson et al 1996). Thus, decreased norepinephrine and cortisol levels and increased serotonin levels were expected following the massage therapy study.

## Results

**Immediate-effects measures (pre/post-therapy sessions)** Analyses conducted on the pre/post measures to assess the immediate effects of the first and last day massage therapy sessions yielded effects suggesting that on both days the massage versus the standard treatment group (see Table 4.8):

1. reported lower anxiety
2. reported less depressed mood
3. were observed to show less anxiety
4. were observed to have more positive affect.

**Table 4.8**  Means for pre/post massage/control[1] measures from first and last day's treatment (Study 4)

|  | First day | | Last day | |
| --- | --- | --- | --- | --- |
|  | Pre | Post | Pre | Post |
| Depressed mood (POMS) | $33.1_a$ | $25.9_b$**** | $27.0_a$ | $18.6_b$**** |
|  | 34.1 | 39.7 | 38.2 | 35.3 |
| Anxiety (STAI) | $50.1_a$ | $39.1_b$**** | $49.1_a$ | $37.4_b$**** |
|  | 57.1 | 55.0 | 55.2 | 54.2 |
| Observed anxiety | $1.7_a$ | $1.2_b$*** | $1.3_a$ | $1.1_a$ |
|  | 1.9 | 1.8 | 1.4 | 1.5 |
| Saliva cortisol (ng/ml) | $1.4_a$ | $1.0_b$* | $0.9_a$ | $0.8_a$ |
|  | 1.2 | 1.4 | 1.0 | 1.2 |

[1] Control means are in the lower row of each pair of rows.
* $p < 0.05$; ** $p < 0.01$; *** $p < 0.005$; **** $p < 0.001$.

**Longer-term effects (first-day/last-day measures)** Analyses of the first-day/last-day measures assessing the longer-term effects of repeated massages yielded effects suggesting (see Table 4.9):

1. improved eating disorder attitudes, including drive for thinness, bulimia, body dissatisfaction, ineffectiveness, perfectionism, interpersonal distrust, interoceptive awareness and maturity fears
2. reported decrease in depression
3. an increase in dopamine levels
4. a decrease in cortisol levels.

## Discussion

Both self-report and behavior observations revealed an immediate decrease in anxiety and depression in these bulimic women after the first and last massage sessions. It was surprising, therefore,

**Table 4.9** Means for first and last day measures for massage and control group[1] (Study 4)

| Measure | First day | Last day |
|---|---|---|
| *Self-report measures* | | |
| Body Scale | | |
|   Body areas | $2.6_a$ | $2.9_b$** |
| | $2.4$ | $2.2$ |
|   Overall appearance | $2.4_a$ | $3.1_b$*** |
| | $2.0$ | $2.2$ |
|   Weight preoccupation | $3.9_a$ | $3.3_b$* |
| | $3.8$ | $3.5$ |
|   Subjective weight | $3.3_a$ | $3.0_b$* |
| | $3.1$ | $2.9$ |
| Eating Disorder Inventory | $87.6_a$ | $48.7_b$**** |
| | $81.2$ | $82.7$ |
| Depression (CESD) | $36.2_a$ | $27.2_b$**** |
| | $38.8_a$ | $30.9_b$* |
| Tactile sensitivity | $29.9_a$ | $21.0_b$* |
| | $27.1$ | $26.9$ |
| *Biochemical measures* | | |
| Self-esteem | $29.7_a$ | $32.7_b$* |
| | $26.9$ | $28.0$ |
| Norepinephrine | $21.7_a$ | $24.9_a$ |
| | $32.3$ | $24.3$ |
| Epinephrine | $5.1_a$ | $4.3_a$ |
| | $8.3$ | $5.7$ |
| Dopamine | $146.5_a$ | $210.8_b$* |
| | $183.0$ | $250.1$ |
| Urinary cortisol | $222.4_a$ | $152.2_b$* |
| | $162.1$ | $140.4$ |

[1] Control means are in the lower row of each pair of rows.
* $p < 0.05$; ** $p < 0.01$; *** $p < 0.005$; **** $p < 0.001$.

that the saliva cortisol levels did not decrease after those sessions. However, the levels were already very low at baseline, probably because sampling occurred late afternoon when cortisol levels typically reach their lowest in the diurnal cycle, making it difficult to decrease further, yet the significant decrease in basal salivary cortisol levels seen from the first to last day and clearly reflected in the marked decrease in the 24-hour urinary cortisol level suggests a significant decrease in stress.

The significant decreases in urinary and salivary cortisol levels by the last day of the study, again, suggests a significant decrease in stress. Again, the convergence of measures, in this case the reported decrease of depression and the decrease in cortisol, is consistent with the behavioral findings. Nonetheless, their depression levels remained high, as might be expected since bulimia is considered a depressive disorder (Edelstein et al 1989). More intensive longer-term massage therapy might be needed to further decrease depression. The significance of the increased dopamine levels is less clear, although dopamine levels are often lower in depressed adults. Although serotonin increased 30% (Kaye et al 1984), this effect was not significant, and norepinephrine did not decrease (Robinson et al 1985, Smythe et al 1983).

Whether decreased depression contributed to improved attitudes regarding their eating disorder, or the improved attitudes contributed to less depression, is also unclear. Direction of effects would of course be difficult to determine. Massage therapy in any case may have raised the patients' awareness of their bodies, which some have said is critical for resolving body perception dissonance (Vandereycken & Meermann 1984).

Although more extensive studies are needed, these data suggest that massage therapy was an effective adjunct to the women's standard treatment. Since anxiety, depression, neuroendocrine abnormalities, and poor self-image are major symptoms of this eating disorder, and since massage therapy attenuated these problems, it would appear to be a treatment of choice for bulimia patients.

## Study 5: Anorexia symptoms are reduced by massage therapy

Anorexia nervosa is diagnosed as body weight 15% below normal in individuals who are fearful of weight gain despite being underweight, disturbed over their body weight or shape, and, among females, if there are disruptions in the menstrual cycle resulting in amenorrhea (American Psychiatric Association 1996). With the rapid growth in cultural expectations that women's bodies should be very thin (Wiseman et al 1992), concerns about body shape and eating emerge as early as adolescence (Bunnell et al 1992, Mueller et al 1995) and may contribute to the 'almost epidemic rise' in the incidence of eating disorders (Wiseman et al 1992, Waltos 1986), now striking 1% of adolescent females and resulting in death in 2–10% of cases (American Psychiatric Association 1996).

Women who have anorexia consistently report comorbidity of eating and affective disorders (Steiger et al 1992), and high depression and anxiety levels are observed in these women (Fornari et al 1992). Eating disorders also affect body image (Cash & Pruzinsky 1990). For example, one study found that dysphoria significantly covaried with women's negative evaluations of their bodies (Denniston, Roth & Gilroy 1992), and, in another study, mood and eating symptoms were linked to body-image concerns, perfectionism, impulsivity, self-criticism, and perceptions of anorexic families as incohesive (Steiger et al 1992).

Due to limited food intake, anorexic individuals can experience biochemical changes, including electrolyte imbalances as well as renal and liver dysfunction (Turner & Shapiro 1992). The energy requirements of the body can shift into a catabolic state in which energy is released through the breakdown of materials in the body, including muscle and other structural proteins, to provide glucose. The production of glucose from alternative substrate sources has been associated with increased cortisol levels, with higher cortisol levels being associated with lower body weight (Turner & Shapiro 1992) and depression (Faustman et al 1990).

Anorexic individuals do not respond readily to treatment (Herzog et al 1992). Recent reviews on the status of treatments for eating disorders (Herzog et al 1992) report that encouraging findings on treatments for bulimia have not been matched in parallel studies on anorexia, with the exception of one study (Halmi et al 1986) which found that the tricyclic antidepressant cyproheptadine was marginally associated with decreases in anorexia symptoms. Psychotherapy has had limited success with outpatients (Hall & Crisp 1987), and studies on inpatients suggest that anorexia is often a chronic condition requiring repeated hospitalization (Szmukler 1985). One study on a clinical population reported that almost one half of inpatients with a diagnosis of anorexia were readmitted to a psychiatry unit within 5 years (McKenzie & Joyce 1992), and another study on a nonclinical population reported that women's scores on the Eating Disorder Inventory (EDI) (Garner et al 1983) were highly stable over a 1-year period (Crowther et al 1992).

Anorexic individuals also report a strong desire for more tactile nurturance. Compared with a nonclinical sample, anorexics have reported greater touch deprivation during their current lives as well as their childhood (Gupta et al 1995). These studies suggest that the inclusion of positive touch experiences such as massage therapy may be important for successful treatment. Studies have shown that elderly individuals (Fakouri & Jones 1987) and hospitalized depressed children (Field et al 1992) showed decreased anxiety, depression, and stress hormones following massage. Bulimic adolescents have also benefitted from massage therapy (Field et al 1998). Massaged patients reported improved attitudes on the Eating Disorder Inventory, including drive for thinness, bulimia, body dissatisfaction, ineffectiveness, perfectionism, interpersonal distrust, interoceptive awareness, and maturity fears. Additionally, they reported lower depression and anxiety levels and they exhibited less anxious behavior and more positive affect. Following a month of treatment, massaged subjects showed lower cortisol, again suggesting reduced stress, and increased dopamine. The present study investigated the effectiveness of massage therapy for women with anorexia nervosa.

## Method

**Sample** Nineteen females (mean age = 25.7) currently undergoing treatment for anorexia were randomly assigned to a massage therapy ($N$ = 10) or a standard treatment only control group ($N$ = 9). Participants' body mass index (BMI = weight in kg/square of height in meters) suggested body weight at least 15% below the normal range (mean = 17.8). Six of the 10 participants in the massage therapy group and 5 of the 9 subjects in the control group were inpatients at a center for eating disorders. Outpatient subjects were recruited from college treatment centers serving women with eating disorders. The inpatients and outpatients did not differ on the BMI, the EDI, or demographic variables (Table 4.10). Subjects in the massage and control groups also did not differ on BMI, EDI, or the demographic variables.

### Treatment procedures

*Massage therapy.* The massage therapy subjects received a 30-minute massage 2 days per week for 5 weeks, for a total of 10 massages. The massage covered the entire body, including 15 minutes in a supine position and 15 minutes in a prone position. In the supine position, four regions of the body were massaged as follows:

1. *head/neck*:
   (a) traction of the neck

**Table 4.10**  Demographics of massage and control group participants (Study 5)

| Variables | Groups | | |
|---|---|---|---|
| | Massage (*N* = 10) | Control (*N* = 9) | *p* |
| Body Mass Index (mean) | 17.4 | 18.3 | NS |
| Age (mean) | 24.9 | 26.3 | NS |
| CES-D (mean) | 39.9 | 35.0 | NS |
| Eating Disorders | | | NS |
|    Inventory (mean) | 88.8 | 83.1 | NS |
|    Inpatients (#) | 6 | 5 | NS |
|    Outpatients (#) | 4 | 4 | NS |

   (b) stroking each side of the neck from head to shoulder with flats of the hands

   (c) with both palms on forehead, stroking outward toward temples

   (d) slow elliptical strokes to the jaw joint with finger tips, continuing to stretch the muscle overlying the jaw joint from the cheekbone to the lower jaw region

   (e) with palms of hands on tops of shoulders, pressing down evenly toward the feet

   (f) for 1 minute, pressing with thumbs into the hollow at the top of the shoulders

2. *arms*:

   (a) traction of arms, supporting the elbow and hand, and moving the arm through the natural range of shoulder motion

   (b) squeezing motions to the entire hand and friction movements with thumbs to the palm

   (c) long, slow gliding strokes from the hand to the shoulder seven times

   (d) slow, rounding strokes encircling the shoulder seven times

   (e) squeezing of the fleshy webbing between the thumb and forefinger for 1 minute

   (f) slow strokes from the shoulder to the hand

3. *torso*:

   (a) holding ribs on both sides and rocking rib cage from side to side

   (b) holding one hand on solar plexus and other hand on forehead

4. *legs*:

   (a) traction of legs, holding at ankles with legs close together, pulling legs straight, and then to the left and right

(b) squeezing the foot and friction movements with thumbs on top of the foot, and pressing with thumbs into the soles of the feet
(c) long, slow gliding strokes from the foot to the hip seven times
(d) slow strokes from the hip to the foot.

In the prone position, the legs and back were massaged as follows:

1. *legs*:
   (a) stretching the Achilles tendon
   (b) stroking up the calf from the ankle to knee and squeezing the fleshy part of the calf
   (c) with one hand on the thigh and the knee bent, shaking muscles
   (d) long strokes from the heel to the buttocks
   (e) slow strokes from buttocks to feet
2. *back*:
   (a) with heel of hands pressing into the low back along the vertebral column, stroking towards the sides of the body
   (b) stroking from base of the spine to shoulders and out to arms
   (c) grasping top of shoulders and squeezing
   (d) with sides of both hands, giving friction from top of back to bottom on either side of the back
   (e) squeezing soft tissue on back of the neck: stretching with one hand towards head and other towards upper back
   (f) with heel of hand just above hips, pressing while pushing the back toward feet
   (g) long slow stroking from shoulders to toes twice
   (h) with one hand on lower back and other between shoulder blades, rocking for 20 seconds and then holding still for 1 minute exerting traction.

### Assessment procedures

*Measures of immediate (pre–post) effects.* The following assessments were administered before and after subjects received massage therapy or engaged in regular activity for 30 minutes: (1) *The State Trait Anxiety Inventory (STAI)* (Spielberger et al 1970); (2) *The Profile of Mood States* (POMS) (McNair et al 1971); (3) *saliva cortisol* (Appendix 2A).

*Measures of longer-term (first-day/last-day) effects.* The following assessments were administered on the first and last days of the 5-week study: (1) *The Center for Epidemiological Studies Depression Scale* (CES-D) (Radloff 1977); (2) *The Eating Disorders Inventory* (EDI) (Garner, et al 1983); (3) *urine sample*.

## Results

Group analyses (Table 4.11) revealed that the massage group scores on the STAI and the POMS decreased after the sessions, and their saliva cortisol levels decreased, suggesting an immediate reduction in anxiety and stress hormone levels and an improved mood following the massage sessions.

Analyses of the longer-term measures (Table 4.12) revealed that after the 5-week treatment period the massage group showed decreased EDI scores. Dopamine also increased in the massage group following the five-week treatment period.

## Discussion

The anorexic women in this study reported decreased anxiety and improved mood immediately following the massage therapy sessions. In parallel with the self-report data, decreases in saliva cortisol levels further suggested reduced stress. These findings support previous reports on the benefits of massage therapy for bulimic women (Field et al 1998). The increased dopamine levels and the increased norepinephrine levels were unexpected and certainly warrant further research.

**Table 4.11** Means of measures for immediate effects (low scores are optimal) (Study 5)

|  | Massage | | Control | |
|---|---|---|---|---|
|  | Pre/Post | Pre/Post | Pre/Post | Pre/Post |
| Anxiety (STAI) | $52.3_a/\ 4.1_b$ | $47.3_a/37.0_b$ | $50.2_a/46.5_a$ | $48.8_a/46.1_a$ |
| Mood (POMS) | $39.5_a/28.5_b$ | $30.0_a/20.2_b$ | $32.8_a/31.7_a$ | $29.1_a/25.0_a$ |
| Saliva cortisol | $1.8_a/\ 1.1_b$ | $1.9_a/\ 1.8_a$ | $1.8_a/\ 1.7_a$ | $1.7_a/\ 1.7_a$ |

Subscripts denote differences between means at $p < 0.05$, contributing to significant group-by-session interactions.

**Table 4.12** Means of measures of longer-term (1-month) effects (Study 5)

|  | Massage | | Control | |
|---|---|---|---|---|
|  | First day | Last day | First day | Last day |
| Eating Disorder Inventory | $88.8_a$ | $66.0_b$ | $83.1_a$ | $80.5_a$ |
| *Urinary assays* |  |  |  |  |
| Dopamine | $146.2_a$ | $252.2_b$ | $176.3_a$ | $166.7_a$ |
| Norepinephrine | $29.2_a$ | $38.1_b$ | $34.7_a$ | $29.8_a$ |
| Epinephrine | $7.9_a$ | $7.5_a$ | $7.5_a$ | $8.9_a$ |
| Cortisol | $172.5_a$ | $155.3_a$ | $211.5_a$ | $188.5_a$ |

Subscripts denote differences between means at $p < 0.05$, contributing to significant group-by-session interactions.

By the last day of the study, the massaged women reported less body dissatisfaction on the Eating Disorder Inventory. That the EDI scores of subjects in the control group were unchanged, despite being in standard treatment, supports reports on the stability of EDI responses (Crowther et al 1992) and confirms observations that anorexia does not respond readily to traditional therapies (Herzog et al 1992). The massage therapy may have been more successful because of the desire for tactile nurturance in anorexic women (Gupta et al 1995). Further studies are needed to explore associations between body satisfaction, the need for tactile nurturance, and massage therapy. By helping women feel more comfortable with their bodies, massage therapy may have facilitated close physical contacts in intimate relationships, thereby satisfying the need for tactile nurturance. Continued research is needed to determine the relationship between body image and the need for tactile nurturance among anorexic women receiving massage therapy.

# CHRONIC FATIGUE

## Study 6: Chronic fatigue syndrome symptoms are reduced by massage therapy

Chronic fatigue immunodeficiency syndrome is a disease whose exact cause is unknown. Its most common symptom is sustained or periodic fatigue which is disproportionate to the patient's exertion and is incapacitating. In addition to the strong evidence of a psychiatric component to chronic fatigue syndrome, recent studies on these patients suggest immune dysfunction. Thus, the true etiology remains elusive. Regardless of its etiology, treatment remains problematic, as therapeutic agents and physical modalities have not successfully reduced the syndrome. The focus of this study was to examine the effects of massage therapy on the wellbeing of patients with chronic fatigue immunodeficiency syndrome. Massage therapy was expected to reduce depression, anxiety, and stress hormones (including cortisol levels and norepinephrine) as it has before in other groups of depressed individuals.

*Method*

**Subjects** Twenty subjects with chronic fatigue immunodeficiency syndrome were recruited from referrals by local physicians. They were randomly assigned to either the massage therapy or an attention control (sham Transcutaneous Electrical Stimulation) group based on a stratification procedure to ensure matched samples.

Ten patients were assigned to each group. The sample was comprised of 80% women and 20% men (mean age = 47). The sample was primarily middle SES (mean = 3.0 on the Hollingshead Index), 80% of the sample was White and 20% Hispanic, 55% were married, 85% were college graduates, 30% were employed, and 56% of the sample had never had a massage. The groups did not differ on these demographic factors, and throughout the study the groups received equivalent therapy contact.

**Treatment procedures** Both groups of subjects were told that these treatments (massage therapy and TENS) were expected to reduce their symptoms. Although the examiners were blind to the group assignment of the subjects, this potential bias would not have affected the data, because the data were collected via self-report measures and biochemical samples. Both the massage therapy and the attention control (sham TENS) subjects participated in treatment sessions in the same laboratory room for the same frequency and intensity (same duration of time at the same intervals). The therapists were asked not to talk with the subjects or in any way display differential treatment aside from the different type of touching. The subjects were assessed on the first day and again 5 weeks later on the last day of the study. On both the first and last day of treatment all subjects were asked to complete the Profile of Mood States, State Anxiety Inventory, and Visual Analogue Scale for Pain before and after their therapy sessions. These scales were used to assess immediate changes in depressed mood, anxiety, and pain after receiving massage therapy.

*Massage therapy.* The massage therapy was given twice a week for 5 weeks by a trained massage therapist and consisted of gentle pressure to the arms, torso, legs, and head. For the first 15 minutes the massage was performed in the face-up position, and for the last 15 minutes it was administered face-down. The massage began with lengthening and stretching of the neck and spine with the hands positioned under the head and neck. This procedure was followed by stroking of the forehead and face. Gentle pressure was applied to the tender points, and the shoulders were then gently depressed. The arms and legs were stretched, and the arms were lifted and moved in a slow circular motion. Light finger pressure was applied to the palms of the hands and the soles of the feet using short, smooth strokes with extra pressure given to the tender points. Medium pressure was administered to the upper shoulder and neck area, while light, brisk rubbing movements were performed along the spine.

*Control group (sham TENS).* The sham TENS group was included in order to control for the attention and tactile stimulation provided by the therapist. The Electro-Acuscope® (a microcurrent transcutaneous electrical nerve stimulator featuring metallic roller probes) was used for the tactile stimulation but was never turned on, so that the subject simply received tactile stimulation (no electrical current) from the roller. The roller probes were rolled back and forth by the therapist over the same body parts that were massaged in the massage group for the same periods of time.

### Assessment procedures

*Assessments of immediate effects (pre and post treatment sessions on first and last days).* These included: (a) *Profile of Mood States* (POMS) (McNair et al 1971); (b) *STAI* (Spielberger et al 1970); (c) *Visual Analogue Scale* (VAS); and (d) *salivary cortisol* (Appendix 2A).

*Assessments of longer-term effects (prior to treatment on the first and last days)*

1. *Center for Epidemiological Studies Depression Scale* (CES–D) (Radloff 1977).
2. *Profile of Fatigue-Related Symptoms (PFRA)* (Ray et al 1992). This questionnaire was specifically designed for patients with CFS. Three subscales were used: fatigue (12 items), emotional distress (15 items), cognitive distress (12 items) and somatic symptoms (16 items).
3. *Pain and Sleep Questionnaire.*
4. *Dolorimeter.* This instrument was used by the rheumatologist (who was blind to the subjects' group assignment) to verify tender points and pain threshold. Point pressure threshold was measured by exerting a force of 1 kg/s over the tender points.
5. *Urine samples for catecholamines and cortisol.*

## Results

**Pre/post-therapy measures** Although depression and anxiety scores were initially as high as they are for clinically depressed patients, analyses of the pre- vs post-therapy measures on the first and last day of treatment revealed that immediately following massage therapy the subjects' depression, pain, and cortisol levels decreased significantly more in the massage therapy than in the sham TENS group (Table 4.13). Although anxiety decreased for both groups, the decrease was significantly greater for the massage therapy group. The pre- and post-treatment measures taken on the last day of therapy also changed significantly more for the massage therapy versus the control group, including greater decreases for depression scores, anxiety scores, pain score ratings, and the salivary cortisol levels.

The massage therapy group values also changed more significantly than the sham TENS group values when the baseline values on the last day were compared with those values from Day 1. The depression scores, the Profile of Fatigue Symptoms scores (fatigue and somatic symptoms), and the Pain and Sleep Symptoms scores improved (pain ratings decreased and hours of sleep increased). The massage group versus the sham TENS also experienced more significant decreases in cortisol levels and increases in dopamine.

### Discussion

The results of this study suggest more significant improvement in self-report measures and biochemical values in those receiving massage versus sham TENS. Depression, anxiety, and pain not only decreased immediately after receiving the first massage but continued to decrease over the 5-week treatment period as shown by the last day versus first day comparisons.

Massage therapy helped alleviate not only fatigue symptoms but other somatic symptoms associated with chronic fatigue immunodeficiency syndrome. The underlying mechanism for this improvement is unclear. As in other studies on massage therapy, the treatment appeared to reduce stress levels (decreased urinary cortisol levels) and enhance sleep, which might explain the reduc-

**Table 4.13** Raw mean scores for massage therapy (T) and sham TENS control (C) group (Study 6)

| Variables | First day | | Last day | |
|---|---|---|---|---|
| | T | C | T | C |
| Depression (CES-D) | 22.8 | (27.6) | 14.8**** | (26.6) |
| Profile of fatigue symptoms | | | | |
| fatigue | 54.8 | (53.4) | 47.6* | (59.6) |
| emotional distress | 34.6 | (43.6) | 23.2**** | (25.0)* |
| cognitive distress | 37.7 | (35.8) | 31.4 | (32.5) |
| somatic symptoms | 37.2 | (43.6) | 27.4*** | (40.7) |
| Pain and sleep symptoms | | | | |
| pain past week | 4.1 | (5.0) | 2.8* | (6.6) |
| # hours of sleep | 6.8 | (6.5) | 7.5* | (6.2) |
| dolorimeter (kg/sec) | 11.4 | (9.0) | 11.9 | (8.0) |
| Biochemical values (ng/mg creatinine) | | | | |
| Norepinephrine | 48.6 | (36.6) | 49.7 | (30.6) |
| Epinephrine | 11.3 | (6.5) | 9.5 | (3.4) |
| Dopamine | 200.7 | (121.2) | 254.1* | (117.7) |
| Cortisol | 164.0 | (183.9) | 96.9*** | (109.5) |

Asterisks next to after session values indicate pre–post session comparisons. Asterisks next to before session values on last day indicate first–last day comparisons: * $p < 0.05$; ** $p < 0.01$; *** $p < 0.005$; **** $p < 0.001$.

tion in chronic fatigue symptoms. The fact that the sham TENS group showed less change during the 5-week study suggests that human touch or deeper pressure than that produced by the TENS roller may be required

Future research in this field is needed. Outcome parameters should include additional measures of fatigue as well as parameters of immune function. Examples include activity bracelets recording the subjects' activity levels, or time lapse videotaping of night-time sleep. In addition, serotonin levels and natural killer cell activity should be measured to quantify improvement in immune function. In the interim, massage therapy appears to be a cost-effective way of reducing symptoms associated with this syndrome and should be seriously considered as a treatment component for those affected by this problem.

## MECHANISMS UNDERLYING TOUCH THERAPY'S REDUCTION OF DEPRESSION

Depressed mood, anxiety levels, and stress hormones were reduced in all of the above studies. One potential mechanism is suggested by a recent study measuring frontal EEG activation following massage in depressed adolescents (Jones & Field in press). Shifts to a more positive mood were notably accompanied by shifts from right frontal EEG activation (normally associated with sad affect) to left frontal EEG activation (normally associated with happy affect) or at least to symmetry (midway between sad and happy affect). In our study on depressed adolescent mothers and their infants, right frontal EEG activation (noted in chronically depressed adults and also observed in the depressed mothers and infants in our study) was shifted towards symmetry following a 20-minute massage. Chemical and electrophysiological changes from a negative to a positive balance may underlie the decrease in depression noted following massage therapy.

A related potential mechanism may be the increase noted in vagal activity following massage therapy. One branch of the vagus (the 'smart' vagus) stimulates facial expressions and vocalizations, which would contribute to less flat facial and vocal expressions; the latter could then feed back to reduce depressed feelings and stress hormones.

In all of these studies, depression, anxiety, and stress hormones significantly decreased following massage therapy. Because depression, anxiety, and stress hormones (particularly cortisol) are notably elevated in autoimmune and immune disorders, we hypothesized that massage therapy might also reduce these problems.

REFERENCES

Adams PR, Adams GR 1984 Mount Saint Helena's ashfall: evidence for a disaster stress reaction. American Psychology 39:252–260
American Psychiatric Association 1987. Diagnostic and statistical manual of mental disorders, 3rd edn. APA, Washington, DC
American Psychiatric Association 1996 Diagnostic and statistical manual of mental disorders 4th edn. APA, Washington, DC
Beck AT, Ward CH, Mendelson M, Mock J, Erbaugh J 1961 An inventory for measuring depression. Archives of General Psychiatry 4:561–571
Bloch DA, Silber E, Perry SE 1956 Some factors in the emotional reactions of children to disaster. American Journal of Psychiatry 133:416–422
Brotman AW, Herzog DB, Woods SW 1984 Antidepressant treatment of bulimia: the relationship between binging and depressive symptomatology. Journal of Clinical Psychiatry 45:7–9
Bunnell D, Cooper P, Hertz S, Shenker IR 1992 Body shape concerns among adolescents. International Journal of Eating Disorders 11:79–83
Burke JD, Borus JF, Burns BJ, Millstein K, Beaslet M 1982 Changes in children's behavior after a natural disaster. American Journal of Psychiatry 139:1010–1014
Cash T, Pruzinsky T 1990 Body images: development, deviance and change. Guilford Press, New York
Cohen J 1968 Weighted kapa: nominal scale agreement provision for scaled disagreement or partial credit. Psychological Bulletin 70:213–220
Cohn JF, Campbell SB, Matias R, Hopkins J 1990 Face-to-face interactions of postpartum depressed and non-depressed mother–infant pairs at two months. Developmental Psychology 26:185–193
Corder B, Whiteside R, Haslip T 1986 Biofeedback, cognitive training and relaxation technique as a model adjunct therapy for hospital aides: a pilot study. Adolescence 21:339–346
Costello EJ, Edelbrock CS, Costello AJ 1985 Validity of the NIMH Diagnostic Interview Schedule for children: a comparison between psychiatric and pediatric referrals. Journal of Abnormal Child Psychology 13:579–595
Crowther J, Lilly R, Crawford P, Shepherd K 1992 The stability of Eating Disorder Inventory. International Journal of Eating Disorders 12:97–101
Denniston C, Roth D, Gilroy F 1992 Dysphoria and body image among college women. International Journal of Eating Disorders 12:449–452
Dohrenwend BP, Dohrenwend BS, Warheit GJ et al 1981 Stress in the community: a report to the President's Commission on the accident at Three Mile Island. Annals of the New York Academy of Sciences 365:159–174
Edelstein CK, Haskew P, Kramer JP 1989 Early cues to anorexia and bulimia. Patient Care 23:155–175
Fakouri C, Jones P 1987 Relaxation therapy: slow stroke back rub. Journal of Gerontological Nursing 13:32–35
Faustman W, Faull K, Whiteford H, Borchert C, Csernansky J 1990 CSF 5-HIAA, serum cortisol, and age differentially predict vegetative and cognitive symptoms in depression. Biological Psychiatry 27:311–318
Field T 1992 Infants of depressed mothers. Development and Psychopathology 4:49–66
Field T, Reite M 1984 Children's responses to separation from mother during the birth of another child. Child Development 55:1308–1316
Field T, Healy B, Goldstein S, Guthertz M 1990 Behavior state matching in mother–infant interactions of non-depressed vs. depressed mother–infant dyads. Developmental Psychology 26:7–14
Field T, Morrow C, Valdeon C, Larson S, Kuhn C, Schanberg S 1992 Massage reduces anxiety in child and adolescent psychiatric patients. Journal of the American Academy of Child and Adolescent Psychiatry 31:125–131
Field T, Schanberg S, Kuhn C, Fierro K, Henteleff T, Mueller C, Yando R, Burman I. (1998). Bulimic adolescents benefit from massage therapy. Adolescence 33:555–563

Fornari V, Kaplan M, Sandberg D, Matthews M, Skolnick N, Katz J 1992 Depressive and anxiety disorders in anorexia nervosa and bulimia nervosa. International Journal of Eating Disorders 12:21–29

Frederick CJ 1985 Children traumatized by catastrophic situations. In: Eth S, Pynoos RS (eds) Post-traumatic stress disorder in children. American Psychiatric Press, Washington DC, pp 73–99

Galante R, Foa D 1986 An epidemiological study of psychic trauma and treatment effectiveness in children after a natural disaster. Journal of the American Academy of Child Psychiatry 25:357–363

Garfinkel PE, Moldofsky H, Garner DM 1977 The outcome of anorexia nervosa, significance of clinical features, body image, and behavior modification. In: Vigersky RA (ed) Anorexia nervosa. Raven Press, New York, pp 315–330

Garner DM, Olmsted MP, Polivy J 1983 The Eating Disorders Inventory: a measure of cognitive-behavioral dimensions of anorexia nervosa and bulimia. In: Darby PL, Garfinkel PE, Garner DM, Coscina DV (eds) Anorexia nervosa: recent developments in research. Alan R. Liss, New York, pp 173–184

Goldman HH 1988 General psychiatry. Appleton & Lange, Norwalk, CT, p 340

Green A 1983 Dimensions of psychological trauma in abused children. Journal of the American Academy of Child Psychiatry 22:231–237

Green BL, Korol M, Grace MC, Vary MG, Leonard AC, Gleser GC, Smitson-Cohen S 1991 Children and disaster: age, gender, and parental effects on PTSD symptoms. Journal of the American Academy of Child and Adolescent Psychiatry 30:945–951

Gupta M, Gupta A, Schork N, Watteel G 1995 Perceived touch deprivation and body image: some observations among eating disordered and non-clinical subjects. Journal of Psychosomatic Research 39:459–464

Hall A, Crisp AH 1987 Brief psychotherapy in the treatment of anorexia nervosa: outcome at one year. British Journal of Psychiatry 151:185–191

Halmi KA, Eckert E, LaDu TJ, Cohen J 1986 Anorexia nervosa: treatment efficacy of cyproheptadine and amitriptyline. Archives of General Psychiatry 43:177–181

Herzog D, Keller M, Strober M, Yeh C, Pai S 1992 The current status of treatment for anorexia nervosa and bulimia nervosa. International Journal of Eating Disorders 12:215–220

Hosmand L, Helmes E, Kazarian S, Tekatch G 1985 Evaluation of a relaxation training program under medical and nonmedical conditions. Journal of Clinical Psychology 41:23–29

Hsu LKG 1986 The treatment of anorexia nervosa. American Journal of Psychiatry 443:573–581

Ironson G, Field TM, Scafidi F, Kumar M, Patarca R, Price A, Goncalves A, Hashimoto M, Kumar A, Burman I, Tetenman C, Fletcher MA 1996 Massage therapy is associated with enhancement of the immune system's cytotoxic capacity. International Journal of Neuroscience 84:205–218

Jones NA, Field T (In Press) Right frontal EEG asymmetry is attenuated by massage and music therapy. Adolescence

Kaye WH, Ebert MH, Gwirtsman HE 1984 Differences in brain serotoninergic metabolism between bulimic and nonbulimic patients with anorexia nervosa. American Journal of Psychiatry 141:1598–1601

Kuhn C, Schanberg S, Field T, Symanski R, Zimmerman E, Scafidi F, Roberts J 1991 Tactile/kinesthetic stimulation effects on sympathetic and adrenocortical function in preterm infants. Journal of Pediatrics 119:434–440

Lacey GN 1972 Observations on Aberfan. Journal of Psychosomatic Research 16:257–260

Livingood AB, Dean P, Smith BD 1983 The depressed mother as a source of stimulation for her infant. Journal of Clinical Psychology 39:369–375

Lonigan DJ, Shannon MP, Finch AJ, Daugherty P, Taylor CM 1991 Children's reactions to a natural disaster: symptom severity and degree of exposure. Advanced Behavioral Research Therapy 13:135–154

Matthew AM, Gelder MG 1969 Psychophysiological reactions to stress. In: Schneiderman N, Tapp J (eds) Behavioral medicine: the biopsychosocial

Three randomly occurring telephone checks were made regarding the parents' compliance. The sessions comprised two standardized phases. For the first phase, the child was placed in a supine position, and oil was applied to ensure smooth, continuous stroking movements. The parents stroked five regions of the child's body in the following sequence: (1) face, (2) chest, (3) stomach, (4) legs, (5) feet, and (6) arms. For the second phase the child was placed in a prone position and the back was massaged.

**Table 5.1** Demographic variables (Study 1)

| | Groups | |
|---|---|---|
| Variables | Massage ($N = 12$) | Control ($N = 12$) |
| Age in years (mean) | 6.5 | 6.9 |
| Gender – Male (%) | 54.5 | 60.0 |
| Ethnicity (%) | | |
|    Hispanic | 36.4 | 20.0 |
|    Non-Hispanic White | 63.6 | 80.0 |
| Socioeconomic status (mean) | 3.0 | 3.1 |

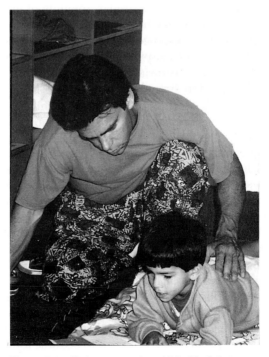

**Figure 5.1** Father massaging child with diabetes.

*Progressive muscle relaxation therapy control group.* The parents in the progressive muscle relaxation group also conducted their sessions in the evenings prior to bedtime for a 4-week period. The parents were trained to ask the child to tense and then to relax each of the same muscle groups in the same sequence of the six body parts that were used in the massage therapy procedure. Thus the relaxation group received the same amount of parent attention time as the massage therapy group and the same number of telephone checks on their compliance.

**Assessments** Pre/post-therapy assessments were made on the first and last days to assess the immediate effects of the two therapies. In addition, first-day/last-day comparisons were made by research assistants who were unaware of the group assignments. These sessions were held at our research laboratory.

*Immediate effects: pre/post therapy on first-day/last-day measures.* The measures were: (1) *STAI* (Spielberger et al 1970); (2) *STAIC* (Spielberger 1973); (3) *Happy Face Scale* (Appendix 3A); (4) *Behavior Observation Ratings* (Platania-Solazzo, et al 1992); (5) *stress hormone (saliva cortisol)*, (Appendix 2A).

*First-day/last-day comparisons (parents' reports).* These included the following.

1. *The Family Environment Scale* (Moos & Moos 1986) includes 90 items that assess 10 domains of family function. For the purpose of this investigation, only the cohesion and conflict domains (18 items) were administered.

2. *The Parenting Stress Index* (Burke & Abidin 1978). For the purpose of this study, two subscales were used: the sense of competence and restriction of role (parental perceptions of being controlled by the demands of the child) subscales. The revised scale includes 18 items rated on a 5-point Likert scale.

3. *The Self Care Inventory* (SCI) (La Greca et al 1990) was completed by the parents, rating the child's typical adherence for 14 regimen behaviors using a 5-point Likert scale. Three subscale scores – blood glucose regulation, insulin, and food regulation and exercise – were used. The SCI has been related to glucose-testing frequency and eating frequency in adults (Greco et al 1990).

4. *Glucose levels.* The children's blood glucose levels were measured by the parents before breakfast each day of the study. The same type of calibrated glucometer (provided by the investigators) was used by all parents, and the parents recorded the values. Although 2–3 other levels were also recorded throughout the day, they were not recorded at the same times across children. Thus,

only the early-morning values were used in this study. Insulin dosages were also recorded by the parents.

## Results

**Pre/post-therapy changes**  Data analyses on the pre/post-therapy changes suggested that the massage therapy group made more positive changes than the relaxation control group (see Table 5.2). Thus, the changes on all of the following measures were significantly greater for the massage therapy group.

1. Parent anxiety (STAI) decreased after therapy on both the first and last days.
2. Child anxiety (STAIC) decreased on both the first and last days.
3. Behavior observation ratings of the children also favored the massage therapy group:
(a) Anxiety decreased on both the first and last days after therapy
(b) Fidgeting decreased on both the first and last days
(c) Affect improved on both the first and last days
4. The children's saliva cortisol levels decreased following therapy on both the first and last days of therapy.

**Table 5.2**  Means for pre/post-massage-therapy (M) and relaxation (R) control groups for first and last day of Study 1 (SDs in parentheses)

| Variables | First day | | | | Last day | | | |
|---|---|---|---|---|---|---|---|---|
| | Pre | | Post | | Pre | | Post | |
| Parent measure | *M* | *R* | *M* | *R* | *M* | *R* | *M* | *R* |
| Parent anxiety (STAI) | 33.6$_a$ | 37.1 | 27.1$_b$** | 32.2 | 32.0$_a$ | 37.0 | 28.1$_b$* | 37.4 |
| | (6.3) | (8.9) | (5.1) | (5.3) | (8.8) | (9.2) | (6.7) | (7.3) |
| *Child measures* | | | | | | | | |
| Child anxiety (STAIC) | 27.9$_a$ | 26.5 | 25.7$_b$* | 27.6 | 31.0$_a$ | 27.5 | 27.3$_b$ | 27.4 |
| | (3.6) | (4.0) | (4.3) | (4.0) | (4.7) | (3.9) | (6.1) | (5.1) |
| Child affect (Faces)[1] | 3.6 | 3.0 | 3.9 | 3.1 | 3.3 | 3.1 | 3.5 | 3.2 |
| | (0.5) | (0.4) | (0.7) | (0.5) | (0.7) | (1.1) | (1.0) | (0.9) |
| Child cortisol (mg/dL) | 1.2 | 1.3 | 0.8[2] | 1.2 | 1.5 | 1.4 | 1.0[1] | 1.5 |
| | (0.6) | (0.7) | (0.5) | (0.5) | (0.5) | (0.7) | (0.5) | (0.6) |
| *Behavioral observations*[1] | | | | | | | | |
| Affect | 2.3$_a$ | 2.2 | 2.9$_b$** | 2.4 | 2.1$_a$ | 2.0 | 3.0$_b$* | 2.3 |
| | (0.5) | (0.4) | (0.5) | (0.6) | (1.0) | (0.9) | (0.0) | (0.9) |
| Anxiety | 1.9$_a$ | 2.0 | 2.8$_b$**** | 2.3 | 2.0$_a$ | 2.0 | 2.8$_b$*** | 2.4 |
| | (0.3) | (0.5) | (0.5) | (0.5) | (0.5) | (0.4) | (1.0) | (0.6) |
| Fidgetiness | 2.0$_a$ | 2.1 | 2.8$_b$*** | 2.4 | 1.9$_a$ | 2.1 | 2.3$_b$** | 2.3 |
| | (0.3) | (0.4) | (0.5) | (0.5) | (0.6) | (0.4) | (1.0) | (0.4) |

[1] Higher scores are optimal.
Different subscript letters indicate significant differences between adjacent columns.
Asterisks indicate level of significance: * $p < 0.05$; ** $p < 0.01$; *** $p < 0.005$; **** $p < 0.001$.

*First-day/last-day changes.* Although the groups did not differ on their first-day pretherapy measures, data analyses suggested changes that were significantly greater for the massage therapy group (see Table 5.3):

1. Cohesion improved on the Family Environment Scale.
2. Sense of competence improved on the Parenting Stress Index.
3. Insulin and food adherence/compliance improved.
4. Blood glucose levels decreased to the normal range – from 158 to 118 (Fig. 5.2). It should be noted that the change in morning glucose values was not inconsistent with changes in values taken later in the day, and by parent records insulin dosages did not change nor were there any severe reactions during the study.

## Discussion

The reduction in parents' anxiety was promising inasmuch as parents with less anxiety have been noted to have children with greater adherence (Mengel et al 1992). Reduced stress in the parents may have contributed to the children's improved insulin and food regulation adherence. Less anxiety (both reported and observed anxiety) and improved affect in the children could

**Table 5.3**   Means for first-day/last-day measures for massage therapy (M) and relaxation (R) control groups (SDs in parentheses) (Study 1)

| Variables | First day | | Last day | |
|---|---|---|---|---|
| *Family environment*[1] | M | R | M | R |
| Cohesion | 7.3$_a$ | 7.0 | 8.7$_b$* | 7.3 |
| | (2.3) | (2.3) | (2.9) | (1.8) |
| Conflict | 1.9 | 1.7 | 1.8 | 1.9 |
| | (1.5) | (1.5) | (1.5) | (1.8) |
| *Parenting stress*[1] | | | | |
| Restriction role | 19.9 | 18.7 | 19.2 | 18.1 |
| | (5.5) | (4.8) | (6.2) | (5.1) |
| Sense of competence | 41.1$_a$ | 49.7 | 51.6$_b$* | 48.6 |
| | (3.7) | (4.6) | (3.0) | (7.1) |
| *Self care inventory*[1] | | | | |
| Glucose regulation | 4.5 | 4.9 | 4.6 | 4.7 |
| | (0.6) | (0.4) | (0.4) | (0.6) |
| Insulin & food regulation | 4.1$_a$ | 4.0 | 4.6$_b$* | 4.1 |
| | (0.7) | (0.7) | (0.5) | (0.6) |
| Exercise | 4.2 | 4.1 | 4.4 | 4.2 |
| | (1.1) | (1.4) | (1.2) | (1.3) |
| *Glucose level*[1] (mg/dL) | 158.7$_a$ | 159.3 | 118.0$_b$* | 147.7 |
| | (50.9) | (57.8) | (29.5) | (44.8) |

[1] Higher means are optimal.
Different subscript letters indicate significant differences between adjacent columns.
Asterisks indicate significant differences between adjacent columns: * $p < 0.05$.

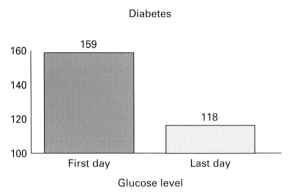

**Figure 5.2** Decrease in blood glucose levels in the massage group of children with diabetes from first to last day of study.

have also contributed to their enhanced compliance, and, in turn, increased adherence and/or lower glucose levels could result in improved affect.

Since 30% of children with diabetes are only partially or inconsistently compliant with recommended diets (Kovacs et al 1992), the improved food and insulin adherence scores following massage therapy are clinically important. Because adherence to insulin and diet are key factors in maintaining metabolic control (Johnson et al 1992), it is perhaps not surprising that the children's blood glucose levels decreased. The 25% decrease in levels more than met the 15% criterion for significant clinical change, and the blood glucose levels moved into the normal range (from 158 to 118, normal range being 70–130).

These data highlight the clinical significance of parents being taught to massage their children with diabetes. In addition to the improvement noted in the children, the parents also experienced decreased anxiety and improved mood, perhaps because they could now contribute to their children's treatment in a more positive way than the typical negative task of testing glucose levels and providing insulin injections.

Assays of glucose levels for the months prior, during, and after the study would have been informative, and values taken at the same time of day and later in the day by all parents would have provided a second test of adherence. In addition, the use of confirmatory measures such as fructosamine and glycosylated hemoglobin, compliance with treatment measures, the children's acceptance of the different therapies, and longer-term follow-up measures, as well as determination of the number of parents who continued the massage therapy after the end of the study would provide more convincing data on the therapeutic value of parents massaging their diabetic children.

# ASTHMA

## Study 2: Pulmonary functions improve in children with asthma after massage therapy

Complementary forms of therapy are being explored for children with asthma. For example, a study on facial relaxation training documented immediate Peak Expiratory Flow Rate (PEFR) increases in children. However, these changes fell short of the standard criterion for clinical significance used in evaluating asthma medication (i.e. a 15% increase in air-flow rates).

Massage therapy was evaluated in the present study because it has effectively lowered anxiety and cortisol levels in children with other problems. Also, it requires less adherence from the children. Another reason for the effectiveness of massage therapy is that the children's parents could provide the therapy. Parents of children with asthma versus parents of children who do not have asthma experience higher anxiety levels which are detrimental to the child's health. Giving the parents an active coping-promoting role in their child's care and therapy may reduce their own anxiety. In addition, a therapy given by parents on a daily basis would be more cost-effective in general.

*Method*

**Sample**   A sample of 32 children with asthma ($N = 16$ massage and 16 control subjects) between the ages 4 and 8 (young group, $N = 16$, mean = 6.2 years) and 9 and 14 years (old group, $N = 16$, mean = 12.1 years) and their mothers were recruited at a pediatric pulmonary clinic. The sample was predominantly lower to middle socioeconomic status (SES) (mean = 3.9 on the Hollingshead Index) with an ethnic distribution of 36% African American, 50% Hispanic, and 14% Non-Hispanic White children, and the mothers averaged 12.2 years education. The children (62% male) had asthma that could be classified as mild for 22%, moderate for 58%, and severe for 20% based on a standardized system (see Measures). In addition, while none of the children experienced emergency admissions to the hospital, 79% had experienced at least one hospitalization in the year preceding the study, while 21% had two hospitalizations during the same period. The children were regularly taking an average of 2.5 different medications (range = 0–6). The children were randomly assigned sequentially to a massage therapy or a

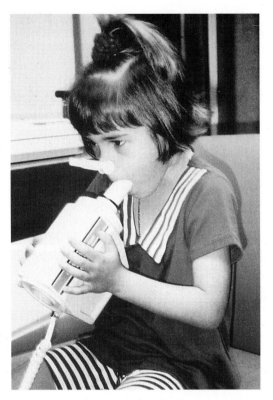

**Figure 5.3** Child with asthma blowing into a peak air flowmeter.

relaxation comparison group based on a stratification procedure to ensure equivalence across groups on age, sex, duration, and severity of condition and medical treatment. The groups did not differ on these variables.

### Procedures

*Massage therapy.* The massage therapy group subjects received a 20-minute massage by their parents just before bedtime every night for 30 days. The parents were given a live demonstration by the massage therapist, written instructions, and a videotaped demonstration to take with them. The massage involved stroking and kneading motions in three regions: (1) face/ head/neck/ shoulders; (2) arms/hands; and (3) legs/feet/back.

*Progressive muscle relaxation therapy comparison group.* This consisted of the parent instructing the child to tense and relax major muscle groups. The same types of parental instruction, duration/ frequency of therapy sessions as those used in the massage therapy group were used for the relaxation group.

**Measures**

*Pre/post-therapy measures taken on the first and last days in the lab to assess immediate effects.* Immediately prior to the therapy session, a saliva sample was collected from the child for cortisol assays as an index of stress reduction. The child's behavior was then videotaped (camcorder on a tripod) during the 30 minutes prior to the therapy and 30 minutes after therapy. The videotapes were subsequently coded by research associates at 30-second time sample units on a 3-point continuum for affect (a global measure of facial expressions, being generally negative or positive), anxiety (fidgeting to relaxed state), and activity (extremes in activity to moderate activity) and vocalizing (negative to positive). The coder was blind to the hypotheses of the study and the group membership of the child. Also, the State Anxiety Scale for the parent and the State Anxiety Scale for Children were completed before and after the sessions because of previous data suggesting that anxiety may be reduced by massage therapy. Thirty minutes following the massage session, another saliva sample was collected from the child.

*First-day/last-day measures to assess longer-term effects.* Asthma severity information was obtained from the parents and Asthma Attitudes (Air Power) from the parents and children. Peak expiratory flow rates were measured using mini-Wright's peak flow meters and were recorded by the parents every night at the same time. Pulmonary function tests were performed on the first and last days of the study using the same spirometer. The following volumes and flow rates were recorded: (a) forced vital capacity; (b) forced expiratory volume in the first second of exhalation; (c) average flow rate measured during the middle half of the forced vital capacity procedure; and (d) peak expiratory flow rate.

*Results*

**Pre/post-therapy-session measures** Data analyses yielded the following immediate effects for the young (4–8 year-old) group (see Table 5.4).

1. The massage versus relaxation children's anxiety levels decreased after the session on the first day, and their activity and vocalization behavior ratings improved after the first and last day massage sessions.

2. The massage versus the relaxation children's salivary cortisol levels decreased on both the first and last days.

For the older children the data analyses revealed the following (see Table 5.5).

1. The parents of both the massage and relaxation children reported lower anxiety levels after the massage on the first day.

2. The massage versus relaxation children reported lower anxiety levels after the massage on the first day.

3. The massage versus relaxation children showed more positive facial expressions after the massage on both the first and last days.

4. The massage versus relaxation children's vocalization ratings improved after the massage on the last day.

**First/last-day measures** Longer-term effects noted for the young group were as follows (see Table 5.6 and Fig. 5.4).

1. The massage versus relaxation children's attitudes toward asthma improved over the 30 days.

2. Their peak air flow ratings taken at home increased over the 30 days.

3. All their pulmonary functions improved including forced vital capacity (a 24% increase), forced expiratory volume (a 27% increase), average flow rate (a 57% increase), and peak expiratory flow rate (a 30% increase).

Longer-term changes over the 30-day period were also noted for the older group (see Table 5.7). However, they were limited to the massage versus relaxation group, showing: (1) greater improvement in their attitudes toward asthma; (2) greater improvement on one measure of pulmonary function – average flow rate increased by 52%.

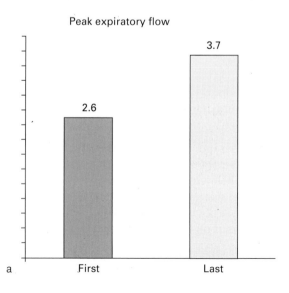

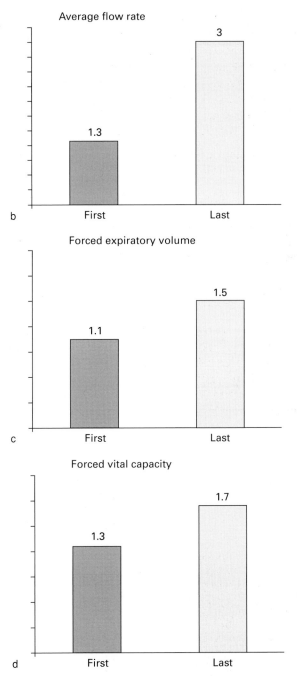

**Figure 5.4**   Improvements in pulmonary functions in young massaged asthmatic group from first to last day of study: (a) peak expiratory flow; (b) average flow rate; (c) forced expiratory volume; (d) forced vital capacity.

**Table 5.4** Means for pre/post measures for young massage and control group (control group is children receiving progressive muscle relaxation therapy) (Study 2)

| | Massage | | Control | |
|---|---|---|---|---|
| | Pre | Post | Pre | Post |
| *Day 1* | | | | |
| Parent anxiety (self-report) | 30.3 | 33.7 | 33.0 | 34.4 |
| Child anxiety (self-report) | 34.7 | 33.5 | 28.0 | 26.0 |
| *Child behavior*[1] | | | | |
| Affect | 2.5 | 2.5 | 2.7 | 3.0 |
| Anxiety | 2.0 | 2.3* | 2.0 | 2.2 |
| Activity | 2.0 | 2.3* | 1.7 | 1.7 |
| Vocalizing | 1.8 | 2.5* | 2.2 | 2.3 |
| Child cortisol (ng/mL) | 1.7 | 1.0*** | 1.2 | 1.2 |
| *Day 30* | | | | |
| Parent anxiety (self-report) | 33.7 | 33.1 | 30.3 | 30.0 |
| Child anxiety (self-report) | 34.0 | 34.2 | 23.0 | 20.7 |
| *Child behavior* | | | | |
| Affect | 2.6 | 2.7 | 3.0 | 3.0 |
| Anxiety | 2.6 | 2.7 | 2.0 | 2.2 |
| Activity | 1.7 | 2.3* | 1.8 | 1.4 |
| Vocalizing | 1.7 | 2.4* | 2.2 | 2.2 |
| Child cortisol | 1.2 | 0.8* | 1.0 | 1.1 |

Asterisks indicate significance of adjacent numbers: * $p < 0.05$; *** $p < 0.005$.
[1] Higher scores are optimal.

**Table 5.5** Means for pre/post measures for older massage and relaxation comparison group (Study 2)

| | Massage | | Relaxation | |
|---|---|---|---|---|
| | Pre | Post | Pre | Post |
| *Day 1* | | | | |
| Parent anxiety (self-report) | 30.5 | 27.6* | 32.2 | 27.6* |
| Child anxiety (self-report) | 32.6 | 28.7* | 30.7 | 34.3 |
| *Child behavior* | | | | |
| Affect | 2.2 | 2.6* | 2.5 | 2.5 |
| Anxiety | 2.0 | 1.8 | 2.0 | 2.3 |
| Activity | 2.3 | 2.6 | 2.0 | 2.2 |
| Vocalizing | 1.9 | 1.9 | 2.0 | 1.5 |
| Child cortisol (ng/mL) | 1.3 | 1.1 | 0.9 | 0.7 |
| *Day 30* | | | | |
| Parent anxiety (self-report) | 30.2 | 29.2 | 32.2 | 27.6 |
| Child anxiety (self-report) | 27.9 | 26.3 | 28.8 | 26.0 |
| *Child behavior* | | | | |
| Affect | 2.1 | 2.9*** | 2.5 | 2.5 |
| Anxiety | 2.3 | 2.6 | 2.0 | 3.0 |
| Activity | 2.1 | 2.4 | 2.0 | 3.0 |
| Vocalizing | 1.7 | 2.3* | 2.0 | 1.5 |
| Child cortisol | 0.8 | 0.9 | 1.2 | 1.6 |

Asterisks indicate significance of adjacent numbers: * $p < 0.05$; *** $p < 0.005$.

## Discussion

The decrease in reported anxiety in the older children and their parents and the decrease from the relatively high baseline saliva cortisol levels in the younger children were promising given that anxiety is noted to exacerbate asthma symptoms. The high level of anxiety typically noted in parents of children with asthma and in the parents of the older children in this study may have been alleviated by teaching them to massage their children.

The peak air flow readings for the young massage children improved as did all of their pulmonary functions. This improvement in clinical condition may have contributed to the young massage children's positive change in attitudes toward asthma. The improved behavior ratings, reduced cortisol levels, and improved pulmonary functions highlight the therapeutic value of

**Table 5.6**  Means for first and last day measures for young massage and relaxation groups (Study 2)

| | Massage (*N* = 16) | | Relaxation (*N* = 16) | |
|---|---|---|---|---|
| | First day | Last day | First day | Last day |
| Children's asthma attitudes | 4.1 | 6.1*** | 5.0 | 5.3 |
| Parents' asthma attitudes | 7.4 | 7.2 | 6.2 | 5.8 |
| Peak flow reading (night before) | 199.3 | 241.4* | 190.0 | 180.8 |
| *Pulmonary functions at lab* | | | | |
| FVC (forced vital capacity) | 1.3 | 1.7** | 1.4 | 1.4 |
| FEV1 (forced expiratory volume) | 1.1 | 1.5** | 1.2 | 1.2 |
| FEF 25–75% (average flow rate) | 1.3 | 3.0*** | 1.4 | 1.6 |
| PEFR (peak expiratory flow) | 2.6 | 3.7*** | 3.1 | 3.2 |

Asterisks indicate significance of adjacent numbers: * $p < 0.05$; ** $p < 0.01$; *** $p < 0.005$.

**Table 5.7**  Means for first and last day measures for older massage and relaxation comparison groups (Study 2)

| | Massage (*N* = 16) | | Relaxation (*N* = 16) | |
|---|---|---|---|---|
| | First day | Last day | First day | Last day |
| Children's asthma attitudes | 6.2 | 7.3*** | 6.7 | 7.0 |
| Parents' asthma attitudes | 5.3 | 6.4 | 5.4 | 5.8 |
| Peak flow reading at home | 334.3 | 49.4 | 302.5 | 292.5 |
| *Pulmonary functions at lab* | | | | |
| FVC (forced vital capacity) | 2.1 | 2.3 | 2.2 | 2.3 |
| FEV1 (forced expiratory volume) | 1.7 | 1.8 | 1.6 | 1.6 |
| FEF 25–75% (average flow rate) | 1.7 | 3.5*** | 1.9 | 2.2 |
| PEFR (peak expiratory flow) | 4.5 | 4.7 | 4.4 | 4.5 |

Asterisks indicate significance of adjacent numbers: *** $p < 0.005$.

massage therapy at least for the younger children with asthma. Although relaxation therapy (progressive muscle relaxation) has also been noted to reduce anxiety and improve peak expiratory flow rate, other pulmonary function measures were not altered by relaxation therapy in these studies or in the present study.

It is not clear why the older children only showed significant improvement in one of the pulmonary functions (average flow rate). Their asthma condition/stress levels may have been worse based on measures that were not recorded in this study. Alternatively, their saliva cortisol levels were within the normal range, having less room to decrease. If massage therapy improves asthma control by reducing the child's anxiety, then the children with the highest baseline anxiety and/or cortisol levels should benefit most from the therapy. Perhaps the older children had less pulmonary function improvement due to their more normal baseline cortisol levels. The older children and their parents might have been less compliant with the therapy protocol, perhaps because they were busier with transition-to-adolescence activities and, thus, less interested in the bedtime massage routine or because they might have felt more awkward about being massaged by their parents even though the massage was essentially a nonintimate backrub. Alternatively, the absence of treatment–control group differences in the older children could have related to the control group using progressive muscle relaxation therapy better than the younger children, resulting in similar effects for the two older groups. Further research will be needed to explore other relaxation techniques for the older children.

In both age groups, there was a significant improvement in average flow rate. This is a sensitive measure of air flow that is thought to reflect primarily flow through small airways. It is relatively effort independent. Since asthma involves small airways, this is an important finding, although the measure reputedly has more intra-individual variability and therefore the actual difference may be less impressive. Daily massage may lead to improved airway tone, decreased airway irritability, and better control of asthma.

A future study would benefit from a diary of asthma episodes and medications to more effectively evaluate the benefits of massage. In addition, it would be important to determine how quickly pulmonary functions improve with massage therapy and whether it might have an even greater impact if it was performed earlier in the day. A longer follow-up period would also be needed to assess the duration of these effects.

# CYSTIC FIBROSIS

## Study 3: Children with cystic fibrosis benefit from massage therapy

Cystic fibrosis (CF) is a chronic, life-threatening disease typically diagnosed in early childhood. The prevalence is about one in 2500 births, making it the most common genetic disease affecting Caucasian children (Thompson et al 1992). CF is characterized by a generalized dysfunction of the exocrine system affecting the gastrointestinal, pancreatic, hepatic, respiratory, and reproductive systems. Chronic lung infections and pancreatic inadequacy, resulting in deficient digestion and malabsorption of nutrients, are the most common complications of this multisystem disease. The mean life expectancy for those with CF has increased due to improved therapies. More than 25% of patients reach adulthood, and 9% live past age 30 (Boucher 1994).

Besides the life-threatening health issues, adjustment problems affect as many as 60% of mothers and 62% of children (Thompson et al 1992). Distress, mild depression, and conduct disorders have been documented (Burke et al 1989, Thompson et al 1992). Unsurprisingly, maternal adjustment has been positively associated with symptom reports (Thompson et al 1992).

Treatment for CF is focused on clearing secretions, controlling infections in the lungs, maintaining nutrition, and preventing intestinal obstruction. Combination therapies include antibiotics to prevent and treat infections, bronchodilators, mucolytics, and corticosteroids (Hodson & Warner 1992), nutritional management that includes pancreatic enzyme supplements (Parker & Young 1991), and physiotherapy (postural drainage) to remove secretions trapped in the airway (Maayan et al 1989). Physiotherapy consists of rhythmic pounding and tapping on different sections of the lungs to facilitate loosening of lung blockage. Typically, parents are trained to administer the physiotherapy. An alternative therapy that has not been explored for children with CF is massage therapy. The relaxing benefits of massage may facilitate coping with CF, as massage has been shown to reduce anxiety, depression, and stress hormones and increase positive affect and cooperative behavior in child and adolescent psychiatric patients (Field et al 1992). In a recent study on asthmatic children, parents were trained to administer massage therapy (Field et al 1998). Pulmonary functions improved, including: peak air flow, forced vital capacity, forced expiratory volume, average flow rate, and peak expiratory flow rate. In addition, children displayed more positive attitudes by the end of the study, and parents' anxiety levels decreased as a result of giving massage therapy.

The present study measured the effects of massage therapy on children with CF as well as their parents. Children receiving the massage were expected to demonstrate less anxiety and depression. Parental anxiety was also expected to decrease from massaging their children. More importantly, the massaged children's peak air flow was expected to improve after a month of massage therapy.

## Method

**Sample** Twenty children with CF ($N$=10 massage and 10 reading control subjects) between the ages of 5 and 15 (mean age = 9.9) were recruited from two cystic fibrosis treatment clinics. The sample was predominantly lower to middle socioeconomic status (mean = 4.1 on the Hollingshead Two Factor Index). Although CF is predominantly a Caucasian disease, because of the ethnic diversity in South Florida, the sample was comprised of 35% Caucasian, 30% African American, and 35% Hispanic. The children's CF condition could be classified as mild for 54%, moderate for 31%, and severe for 15% (see Procedures). Thirty percent were perceived by the parent as getting better, 30% as staying the same, and 40% as getting worse. Forty-two percent of the children had not been hospitalized in the past 12 months, whereas 15% had been hospitalized once, 33% had two hospitalizations, and 10% had more than two hospitalizations in the past year. Subjects were randomly assigned to a massage or control group. The groups did not differ on the above variables.

**Procedures** During the study period, the children continued to receive standard medical care, including examinations by their pulmonary clinic. Zimmerman's system (Zimmerman et al 1987) for assessing severity of asthma in children was modified to assess severity of the CF children in this study, as follows. Level 1 (mild) characterizes children who cough and wheeze intermittently, primarily in the presence of upper respiratory infections. Level 2 (moderate) is characterized by coughing and wheezing in the absence of respiratory infections. Level 3 (severe) requires continuous administration of multiple medications and/or hospitalization.

*Massage therapy.* The children in the massage group received a 20-minute massage from a parent before bedtime every night for 30 days. Parents were given written instructions and trained by a massage therapist on how to conduct the massages. Using small pillows under the legs and hips, the child was first positioned lying on the back at a 45° angle to assist postural drainage. The massage began by stroking with the flats of fingers the

1. *face/head area*:
   (a) strokes to forehead starting from the middle with both hands and then moving towards side of face
   (b) strokes under cheekbones, using fingertips from nose to jaw (under cheekbones) and back
   (c) strokes upwards from middle of jaw to sides of face
   (d) massage to outer ears, bottom to top
   (e) small circles with fingers over entire scalp
2. *neck*: fingertips and flats of fingers in upward strokes from base of neck to base of skull
3. *chest*:
   (a) smooth strokes along the sternum and upper ribs, using flats of fingers and palms
   (b) strokes from waist to shoulder along the side of body
4. *abdomen*: following the colon,
   (a) circular, clockwise strokes over the abdomen
   (b) flat, gliding clockwise strokes over the abdomen
   (c) strokes to the sides of the trunk, from waist up to the shoulder
5. *arms*:
   (a) short and long strokes with thumbs to top of hand and then to palm
   (b) long gliding strokes from wrist to shoulder
   (c) rolling arm from wrist to shoulder, using flats of hands
6. *front of legs*:
   (a) long strokes from ankle, to outside at hip and back down to foot, first using one hand and then using both hands to deliver strokes
   (b) small circles over the knee
7. *foot*:
   (a) strokes, using thumbs, to work top of foot from ankle to toes,
   (b) circles and criss-cross strokes, using thumb, to bottom of foot
   (c) squeezes and light pulls to each toe.

With the child face down
8. *back*:
   (a) criss-cross strokes, with flats of hands, from waist to neck
   (b) small circles, using fingertips, along side of spine from neck to waist

  (c) strokes with flats of hands from spine to side, starting at waist and moving up to neck and back down
  (d) strokes down back from neck to waist, using flats of hands
9. *back of legs*:
  (a) strokes on outside of legs from ankle to hip
  (b) circular movements, using thumbs, to back of knee
  (c) large circles over back of calf muscle, moving from ankle to knee, and then flat strokes moving back and forth to ankle
  (d) continuous circles around the ankles
  (e) large circles over bottom of foot, using thumbs
  (f) shaking/rocking of leg.

*Control group.* Parents of children in the control group were instructed to read to the child for 20 minutes prior to bedtime. This controlled for potential placebo effects that might be attributed to attention from a parent.

**Assessments**

*Pre/post-session assessments (immediate effects).* These assessments were made before and after the sessions on the first and last days of the 30-day study: (1) *The STAI and STAIC* (Spielberger et al 1970; Spielberger 1973); (2) *The Profile of Mood States* (POMS) (McNair et al 1971).

*First/last-day assessments (longer-term effects).* These assessments were made on the first and last days of the study: (1) The *CES–D* (Radloff 1977); (2) *peak expiratory flow rates*. The children drew three separate breaths into a pediatric peak flow meter. The three scores were averaged to compute a mean peak expiratory flow rate. This is a simple procedure, and young children can be taught to give reproducible results using peak flow meters.

*Results*

  **Pre/post-session assessments (immediate effects)** Data analyses revealed a reduction in anxiety (lower STAIC scores) following the session on the first day for the parents and both days for the children, and improved mood (higher POMS scores) in the massaged children following the first and last day sessions (see Table 5.8).

  **First-last-day assessments (longer-term effects)** Data analyses suggested:

1. a reduction in the massaged children's anxiety levels on the last day compared with the first day (see Table 5.8)

**Table 5.8** Means for pre/post measures for massage and control (reading) group for first and last day of Study 3

| | Massage | | | | Control | | | |
|---|---|---|---|---|---|---|---|---|
| | First day | | Last day | | First day | | Last day | |
| Measures | Pre | Post | Pre | Post | Pre | Post | Pre | Post |
| *Immediate effects* | | | | | | | | |
| Parent's anxiety (STAI) | 41.1$_a$ | 36.4$_b$** | 29.7$_b$* | 30.9$_b$* | 37.0$_a$ | 35.5$_a$ | 36.3$_a$ | 40.0$_a$ |
| Child scales | | | | | | | | |
| Anxiety (STAIC) | 32.2$_a$ | 26.1$_b$** | 26.1$_b$** | 24.7$_b$** | 30.8$_a$ | 30.2$_a$ | 33.1$_a$ | 32.9 |
| Mood (POMS) | 4.6$_a$ | 2.0$_b$** | 3.6$_a$ | 1.7$_b$* | 5.7$_a$ | 6.4$_a$ | 8.5$_a$ | 7.2$_a$ |

| | Massage group | | Control group | |
|---|---|---|---|---|
| Longer-term effects | First day | Last day | First day | Last day |
| Depression (CES–D) | 9.7$_a$ | 10.3$_a$ | 14.2$_a$ | 11.6$_a$ |
| Peak air flow[1] | 271.5$_a$ | 297.9$_b$** | 255.0$_a$ | 244.0$_a$ |

Asterisks indicate significance levels for adjacent numbers in the case of pre/post-massage-session changes and those appearing in column 3 reflect the differences between pre-massage values on first and last days: * $p < 0.05$; ** $p < 0.01$.
[1] Higher numbers are optimal.

2. low CES–D scores suggesting that the children were not depressed; no changes were observed from the first to the last day of the study
3. an increase in peak air flow readings for the massage group by the last day of the study (see Table 5.8).

## Discussion

The immediate effects of massage therapy for children with cystic fibrosis included reduced anxiety levels and improved mood. The children's self-report of decreased anxiety persisted over the course of the month, suggesting a longer-term effect. These data are consistent with our recent study showing decreased anxiety in children with asthma (Field et al 1998). The reduced anxiety in the parents (at least after the first session) is promising in that studies show that decreased maternal anxiety facilitates child adjustment to cystic fibrosis (Thompson et al 1992).

The increased peak air flow readings following 1 month of massage therapy are encouraging since these tests correlate well with other assessments of airway obstruction. The peak air flow increase in the CF children is also consistent with the increases reported for children with asthma (Field et al 1997). Future studies might explore longer-term effects of massage on pulmonary functions. Daily massage over 3 months, for example, may lead to improved airway tone and decreased irritability due to vigorous coughing and physiotherapy (Hodson & Warner 1992). In addition, massage therapy may be helpful in alleviating some of the gastrointestinal symptoms experienced by children with CF, such as abdominal pain and weight loss (Stark et al 1993) inasmuch as massage therapy has reduced pain and enhanced weight gain in other studies (Field 1998).

In sum, the findings from this research suggest that massage is an effective treatment for both the receiver and giver. Children with cystic fibrosis benefitted from reduced anxiety, improved mood, and increased peak air flow following massage therapy. Parents who massaged their children also experienced reduced anxiety. Also, because parents can be easily taught to massage their children on a daily basis, this form of therapy can be considered a cost-effective treatment.

# DERMATITIS

## Study 4: Atopic dermatitis symptoms decreased in children following massage therapy

In a pediatric dermatology clinic study, Schachner and his colleagues (1983) reported that atopic dermatitis (AD) was the leading diagnosis for 456 out of 1578 children, exceeding the second most diagnosed disorder, impetigo, by 292 patients. The frequency of AD is still increasing. One recent study indicates that some form of atopy (AD, hayfever, or asthma) occurs in 22.5% of the general population.

The severity of atopic dermatitis has been correlated with depression, stress, and anxiety, which probably cause the negative effects on the immune system via stress increasing cortisol levels and cortisol destroying immune cells. The skin has been described as a 'shock organ' for emotional stress, which manifests itself in the form of skin diseases. Stress may lead to increased histamine release, and itchiness results from excess histamines in the skin. Dermatitis symptoms have also been associated with vasoconstriction and reduced skin blood supply in the affected areas of the skin. Under chronic stress the patient encounters peripheral vasoconstriction mediated by the sympathetic nervous system.

Atopic dermatitis can be a source of great mental embarrassment and insecure feelings, particularly for a child who feels 'different' from other children. Feelings of estrangement can heighten the stress and anxiety, which in turn affect the course of the disease. Because there is evidence suggesting that eczema outbreaks and their severity are influenced by psychological stress, some have used stress reduction as a course of treatment.

Although pharmacotherapies are often effective with atopic dermatitis, stress reduction therapies can be a helpful adjunct to pharmacological therapy. The AD condition may improve, and thus the need for medication may decrease (and the cost of treatment decline) following stress reduction therapies. For example, relaxation therapy may reduce the severity of eczema and the irritation associated with the disorder because relaxation exercises interfere with the scratch and itch cycle that worsens the dermopathic condition. Progressive muscle relaxation training and biofeedback have reduced scratching habits in adults and it has reduced stress, anxiety and stress hormones (cortisol) in child psychiatry patients.

Massage therapy might also improve children's dermatitis inasmuch as massage therapy also decreases stress, anxiety and stress hormones (cortisol and norepinephrine) in children. Massage therapy might be more effective than relaxation therapy for atopic dermatitis patients because of the following.

1. It requires less compliance from the children.

2. It would increase peripheral skin blood supply (a putative contributing problem for AD patients).

3. It has been known to increase vagal activity in other massage therapy studies. Increased vagal activity (increased parasympathetic activation) would reduce the peripheral vasoconstriction associated with sympathetic activity.

4. It might decrease itching as it has been noted to do in post-burn patients.

5. Receiving touch therapy might reduce the AD child's awkwardness about being touched.

Although relaxation therapy is usually considered more cost-effective, massage therapy was considered cost-effective in this study because it could easily be administered by parents. The parents would also benefit by performing a socially acceptable form of touching their children and would feel a sense of actively participating in the treatment process. Finally, the parents could perform the massage therapy while applying medications, emollients, and creams and thus facilitate the standard medical care. The children in turn were expected to have less anxious behavior and improved skin conditions.

*Methods*

**Participants** Twenty children (7 females) with atopic dermatitis (range = 2 to 8 years old, mean = 3.8) were recruited from the Dermatology Department. The children were primarily middle socioeconomic status (range = 2–4, mean = 3.2 on the Hollingshead Index), and they were distributed 28% Black, 61% Hispanic, and 11% White. The children were given the diagnosis of AD an average of 2 months previously and had experienced the current flare for an average of 12 months. As judged by the mother, the child's skin condition had impacted on appearance hardly at all in 11% cases, somewhat in 67%, cases and a lot in 22% cases. Eighty-four percent of the children had at least one other allergy, 68% had at least two additional allergies, and one child had as many as 9 other allergies. Sixty-four percent of the children had at least one other family member who was experiencing similar problems. The children were randomly assigned to a standard care control group or a massage group (who continued to receive standard care) based on a stratification of moderate to severe condition, age, and gender. The children were seen twice, on Day 1 and 1 month later.

**Procedures**

*Standard care.* The children continued to receive treatment from a dermatologist consisting mainly of emollients and topical corticosteroids. These included: (1) topical hydrocortisone ointment to the face, groin and trunk twice daily or as needed; (2) aquaphor applied twice daily; (3) age-appropriate doses of Benadryl every 6 hours or as needed; (4) oral antibiotics for superinfection, as needed. Patients who appeared superinfected had their skin and nares cultured. The parents were instructed to keep a log of the medications used.

*Massage therapy.* The massage therapy group patients were given daily 20-minute massages by their parents. During the first session the therapist gave the parents a 20-minute massage to acquaint them with the techniques and how the massage feels. Then the therapists demonstrated the massage techniques on the child. Finally, the parents were given a videotape and a written description of the massage to take home and review. The massage consisted of two standardized phases. During the first phase, the child was placed in a supine position and the standard medication was used as an emollient (instead of oil) to ensure smooth, stroking movements. The parent stroked five regions of the child's body in the following sequence:

1. *face*:
(a) strokes along both sides of the face

(b)  flats of fingers across the forehead
(c)  circular strokes over the temples and the hinge of the jaw
(d)  flat finger strokes over the nose, cheeks, jaw, and chin
2. *chest*:
(a)  strokes on both sides of the chest with the flats of the
    fingers, going from midline outward
(b)  cross strokes on sides of the chest going over the shoulders
(c)  strokes on sides of the chest toward the shoulder
3. *stomach*:
(a)  hand-over-hand strokes in a paddlewheel fashion, avoiding
    the ribs and the tip of the rib cage
(b)  circular motion with fingers in a clockwise direction starting
    at the appendix
4. *legs*:
(a)  strokes from hip to foot
(b)  squeezing and twisting in a wringing motion from hip to foot
(c)  massaging foot and toes
(d)  stretching the Achilles tendon
(e)  gently stroking the legs upward toward the heart
5. *arms*:
(a)  strokes from the shoulder to the hand
(b) the same procedure as for the legs. Any severely affected AD
    areas of the body that were sensitive were avoided.

### Assessments

*Pre/post-therapy session assessments.*  Before and after the procedure on the first and last days of the study, the parents were asked
to complete self-report scales on their anxiety, the child's behavior
was observed, and an age-appropriate measure of mood was given
to the child. These assessments were administered as follows:

(1) STAI (Spielberger et al 1970) to the parents; (2) *The Happy
Face Scale* (Appendix 3A) to the children; (3) *The Behavior Observation
Scale* (Platania-Solazzo et al 1992).

*First-day/last-day assessments*

1. *The Tactile Defensiveness Scale* (Appendix 5A) measures the
child's typical response to touch. Characteristic yes or no items
include, 'Does your child stiffen his/her body when picked up?',
'Does your child dislike being held, cuddled and hugged?' and
'Does your child enjoy playing with other children?' This scale has
adequate validity and discriminates between groups of children
with and without tactile sensitivity.

2. *How I Feel About My Child* (Appendix 5B). This 17-item scale
taps the parents' feelings about the child's wellbeing and taking
care of the child on a 5-point Likert scale.

3. *Dermatological assessment.* The clinical status of the atopic dermatitis was defined both globally and focally (target area) on a scale of 0 to 3 for the parameters of redness, lichenification, scaling, excoriation, and pruritus. These assessments were made by the dermatologist and the dermatology fellow, who were blind to the child's group assignment.

## Results

**Pre/post-session comparisons: children's behavior and parents' anxiety** Data analyses revealed the following effects favoring the massage group (see Table 5.9).

1. The massaged children's affect and activity levels improved and their anxiety decreased, but only on the last day.
2. The parents' reported anxiety levels decreased after the first massage session and by the last day of treatment.

**First-day/last-day comparisons** Data analyses revealed the following (see Table 5.10).

1. The parents' assessment of their child's anxiety and stability improved on the Coping Index.
2. The parents' feeling about (their) child improved.

Data analyses on the skin assessments revealed the following (see Table 5.11).

**Table 5.9** Means for pre/post-session child and parent measures[1] (Study 4)

| Variables | First day | | Last day | |
|---|---|---|---|---|
| | Pre | Post | Pre | Post |
| *Parent measure* | | | | |
| Anxiety (STAI)[2] | 41.5 | 33.3* | 35.3* | 35.9 |
| | 38.9 | 35.6 | 38.8 | 38.5 |
| *Child measures* | | | | |
| Happy Faces | 3.8 | 3.9 | 4.0 | 4.0 |
| | 3.4 | 3.7 | 2.7 | 3.0 |
| *Behavioral observations* | | | | |
| Affect | 2.9 | 2.6 | 2.6 | 3.0* |
| | 2.8 | 2.8 | 2.7 | 2.7 |
| Activity | 1.9 | 2.1 | 1.3 | 1.7* |
| | 1.8 | 1.5 | 2.0 | 2.0 |
| Anxiety | 2.4 | 2.7 | 2.3 | 3.0* |
| | 2.3 | 2.3 | 2.2 | 2.0 |

[1] Means for the control group are in the lower row of each pair of rows.
[2] Lower score is optimal.
* $p < 0.05$.

**Table 5.10**   Means for first-day/last-day parent assessments[1] (Study 4)

|  | First day | Last day |
|---|---|---|
| *Parent assessments* | | |
| Tactile Defensiveness[2] | 4.0 | 3.5 |
|  | 5.2 | 5.1 |
| *Child's Coping Index* | | |
| Anxiety | 4.9 | 6.8** |
|  | 6.1 | 4.4 |
| Soothability | 7.6 | 7.7 |
|  | 5.1 | 6.1 |
| Stability | 6.3 | 7.6* |
|  | 6.3 | 5.2 |
| *Parent's Coping Index* | 42.6 | 43.2 |
|  | 44.7 | 43.3 |
| Feelings About Child | 69.2 | 73.6* |
|  | 67.2 | 67.0 |

[1] Means for the control group are in the lower row of each pair of rows.
[2] Lower score is optimal.
* $p < 0.05$, ** $p < 0.01$.


**Table 5.11**   Means for first-day/last-day children's skin assessments[1] (Study 4)

|  | First day | Last day |
|---|---|---|
| *Focal area*[2] | | |
| Redness | 2.1 | 1.4*** |
|  | 1.5 | 1.4 |
| Lichenification | 1.8 | 0.9* |
|  | 1.7 | 1.7 |
| Scaling | 1.3 | 0.6* |
|  | 1.9 | 1.4* |
| Excoriation | 1.7 | 0.6** |
|  | 1.5 | 1.1 |
| Pruritus | 1.9 | 1.5* |
|  | 1.5 | 1.7 |
| *Global area*[2] | | |
| Redness | 1.6 | 1.4 |
|  | 1.4 | 1.7 |
| Lichenification | 1.4 | 1.2 |
|  | 1.5 | 1.0 |
| Scaling | 1.5 | 0.6* |
|  | 1.9 | 0.9* |
| Excoriation | 1.6 | 1.0* |
|  | 1.5 | 1.1 |
| Pruritus | 1.9 | 1.5 |
|  | 1.4 | 1.7 |

[1] Means for the control group are in the lower row of each pair of rows.
[2] Lower score is optimal.
* $p < 0.05$; ** $p < 0.01$; *** $p < 0.005$.

1. For the *focal area* assessment, redness, lichenification, excoriation, and pruritus improved by the last day of treatment, but only for the massage group. Scaling was the only measure on which both groups showed improvement over the 1-month period.

2. For the *global area* assessment, scaling and excoriation improved for the massage group and only scaling improved for the control group.

## Discussion

The massaged children's clinical condition, particularly for focal area assessments, improved following 1 month of parents giving the children daily massages before bedtime. This improvement occurred for all measures (redness, lichenification, scaling, excoriation, and pruritus) in contrast to the control group, which only improved on the scaling measure. The massage group also showed improvement on the global area assessments but only for the scaling and excoriation (and the control group only for the scaling) measures. These dermatological assessments document significant improvement in the children's clinical condition following a massage therapy regime.

The observed improvements in the children's conditions may have been mediated by massage decreasing anxiety levels in the parents and children. The children's behavior was less anxious, and their affect and activity levels improved. In addition, the parents perceived their children's anxiety levels as having decreased. The parents also reported that their own anxiety levels decreased and their feelings about their children improved. Direction of causality cannot, of course, be determined in this study. However, the data from behavioral and clinical observations of the child, and the parent's observation of the child, converge to suggest that massage therapy has beneficial effects on children with atopic dermatitis.

REFERENCES

Boucher RC 1994 Cystic fibrosis. In: Isselbacher KJ, Martin JB, Braunwald E, Fauci AS, Wilson JD, Kasper DL (eds) Harrison's principles of internal medicine, 13th edn. McGraw-Hill, New York, pp 1194–1197

Burke WT, Abidin RR 1978 The development of a parenting stress index. Paper presented to APA, Division 37, August 1978

Burke P, Myer V, Kocoshis S, Orenstein DM, Chandra R, Nord DJ, Sauer J, Cohen E 1989 Depression and anxiety in pediatric inflammatory bowel disease and cystic fibrosis. Journal of the American Academy of Child and Adolescent Psychiatry 28:948–951

Chase HP, Jackson GG 1994 Stress and sugar control in children with insulin-dependent diabetes mellitus. Diabetes Spectrum 7:32

Delamater AM, Cox DJ 1994 Psychological stress, coping and diabetes. Diabetes Spectrum 7:17–49

Field T, Morrow C, Valdeon C, Larson S, Kuhn C, Schanberg S 1992 Massage reduces anxiety in child and adolescent psychiatric patients. Journal of the American Academy of Child and Adolescent Psychiatry 31:125–131

Field T, Seligman S, Scafidi F, Schanberg S 1996 Alleviating posttraumatic stress in children following Hurricane Andrew. Journal of Applied Developmental Psychology 17:37–50

Field T 1998 Massage therapy effects. American Psychologist 53:1270–1281

Field T, Henteleff T, Hernandez-Reif M, Martinez E, Mavunda K, Kuhn C, Schanberg S 1998 Children with asthma have improved pulmonary function after massage therapy. Journal of Pediatrics 132:854–858

Field T, Hernandez-Reif M, LaGreca A, Shaw K, Schanberg S, Kuhn C 1997 Glucose levels decreased after giving massage therapy to children with diabetes mellitus. Diabetes Spectrum 10:23–25

Field T, Scafidi F, Pickens J et al 1998 Polydrug using adolescent mothers and their infants receiving early intervention. Adolescence 33:118–143

Fisher E, Delamater A, Bertelson A, Kirkley B 1982 Psychological factors in diabetes and its treatment. Journal of Consulting and Clinical Psychology 50:993–1003

Greco P, La Greca AM, Ireland S, Wick P, Freeman C, Agramonte R, Gutt M, Skyler JS 1990 Assessing adherence in IDDM: a comparison of two methods. Diabetes 39:657

Guthrie DW, Sargent L, Speelman D, Parks L 1990 Effects of parental relaxation training on glycosylated hemoglobin of children with diabetes. Patient Education and Counseling 16:247–253

Hanson CL, Hengeller SW, Burghen GA 1994 Social competence and parental support as mediators of the link between stress and metabolic control in adolescents with insulin-dependent diabetes mellitus. Diabetes Spectrum 7:19–25

Helz JW, Templeton B 1990 Evidence of the role of psychological factors in diabetes mellitus: a review. American Journal of Psychiatry 147:1275–1282

Hodson ME, Warner JO 1992 Respiratory problems and their treatment. British Medical Bulletin 48:931–948

Johnson SB, Kelly M, Henretta JC, Cunningham WK 1992 A longitudinal analysis of adherence and health status in childhood diabetics. Journal of Pediatrics 17:537–553

Kovacs M, Goldstein D, Obrosky S, Lyengar S 1992 Prevalence and predictors of pervasive non-compliance with medical treatment among youths with insulin-dependent diabetes mellitus. Journal of the American Academy of Child and Adolescent Psychiatry 31:1112–1119

La Greca AM, Follansbee D, Skyler JS 1990 Developmental and behavioural aspects of diabetes management in youngsters. Children's Health Care 19:132–139

Lammers CA, Naliboff BD, Straatmeyer AJ 1984 The effects of progressive relaxation on stress and diabetic control. Behavior Research and Therapy 2:641–650

Maayan Ch, Bar-Yishay E, Yaacobi T, Marcus Y, Katznelson D, Yahav Y, Godfrey S 1989 Immediate effects of various treatments on lung function in infants with cystic fibrosis. Respiration 55:144–151

McNair DM, Lorr M, Droppleman LF 1971 POMS – profile of mood states. Educational and Industrial Testing Service, San Diego

Mengel MB, Lawler MK, Volk RJ, Vanini NJ 1992 Parental stress response within a family context: association with diabetic control in adolescents with IDDM. Family Systems 10:395–404

Moos RH, Moos BS 1986 Family environment Scale manual. Consulting Psychologists Press, Palo Alto, CA

Parker AE, Young CS 1991 The physiotherapy management of cystic fibrosis in children. Physiotherapy 77:594–586

Platania-Solazzo A, Field T, Blank J, Seligman F, Kuhn C, Schanberg S, Saab P 1992 Relaxation therapy reduces anxiety in child/adolescent psychiatry patients. Acta Paedopsychiatrica 55:115–120

Radloff LS 1977 The CES–D Scale: a self-report depression scale for research in the general population. Applied Psychological Measures 1:385–401

Schachner L, Ling NS, Press S 1983 A statistical analysis of a pediatric dermatology clinic. Pediatric Dermatology 1:157–164

Spielberger CD 1973 State-trait anxiety inventory for children. Consulting Psychological Press, Palo Alto, CA

Spielberger CD, Gorsuch RC, Lushene RE 1970 The State Trait Anxiety Inventory. Consulting Psychologists Press, Palo Alto, CA

Stark LJ, Knapp LG, Bowen AM, Powers SW 1993 Increasing calorie consumption in children with cystic fibrosis: replication with 2-year follow-up. Journal of Applied Behavior Analysis 26:435–450

Stevens JP 1990 Intermediate statistics: a modern approach. Lawrence Erlbaum, Hillsdale, NJ

Surwit RS, Feinglos MN 1983 The effects of relaxation on glucose tolerance in non-insulin dependent diabetes. Diabetes Care 6:176–179

Thompson RJ, Gustafson KE, Hamlett KW, Spock A 1992 Psychological adjustment of children with cystic fibrosis: the role of child cognitive processes and maternal adjustment. Journal of Pediatric Psychology 17:741–755

Tomakowsky J, Delamater AM, Boardway R, Gutai J 1991 Daily stress, emotions and blood glucose levels in diabetic adolescents. Paper presented at the 12th Annual Meeting of the Society of Behavioral Medicine, Washington DC

Zimmerman B, Stringer D, Feanny S et al 1987 Prevalence of abnormalities found by sinus x-ray in childhood asthma, lack of relation to severity of asthma. Journal of Allergy and Clinical Immunology 80:268–273

# 6

# Immune disorders

Because immune and autoimmune disorders both involve dysfunction in the immune system, the same rationale used for hypothesizing massage therapy effects on autoimmune problems was used for immune disorders. While immune cells destroy the body's other cells in autoimmune disorders, the immune cells are destroyed by foreign cells (viral cells) in immune disorders.

## HUMAN IMMUNODEFICIENCY VIRUS
### Study 1: HIV-positive adults

Although the literature does not include articles on the impact of massage on traditional immune measures, the data from relaxation studies may be of some relevance. Progressive relaxation has been associated with significant increases in natural killer (NK) cell activity in adults (Kiecolt-Glaser et al 1985). In combination with stress management techniques, relaxation training has also been associated with increases in NK cytotoxicity and NK cell number in melanoma patients (Fawzy et al 1990). Finally, in an HIV-positive sample, patients who practiced relaxation more frequently had better immune functioning 1 year after receiving news of seropositive status, and slower disease progression 2 years after this news (Ironson et al 1994).

The purpose of the present study was to assess massage therapy effects on HIV patients. Changes in anxiety levels, relaxation and stress hormones were also assessed as possible underlying mechanisms.

*Method*

**Subjects** Twenty-three HIV-positive and 10 HIV-negative men were recruited for the study. After attrition, 20 HIV-positive and nine HIV-negative men completed the month long massage protocol. We recruited gay men who had no AIDS-defining symptoms.

The sample comprised well-educated (two thirds were college graduates), middle socioeconomic status, gay men who averaged 33 years old. Most of our subjects were asymptomatic; 5 of the 23 HIV positive subjects had symptoms previous to the study (one had thrush and shingles, one had shingles, one had thrush and night sweats, one diarrhea and night sweats, and one night sweats alone). Only two of our subjects were on antiretrovirals (both on AZT).

**Procedure**

*Design overview.* The study was conducted in two cohorts. The first cohort (10 HIV-positive and 10 HIV-negative men), received one month of daily 45-minute massages. Biological measures (blood draws and 24-hour urine collections) and psychological questionnaires were obtained before the first massage and at the end of the month of massages. The first cohort contained both HIV-positive and HIV-negative men in case the massages were differentially effective in the two groups. (There were no significant differences in effect for the two groups in this cohort.) Because our preliminary results from this cohort were promising, a second cohort of 13 HIV-positive men underwent the month long massage period.

*Baseline and other measurement sessions.* At the first session subjects delivered their 24-hour urine collection and had their blood drawn. Next, the subjects completed a questionnaire on demographics, a life events scale, the Profile of Mood states (POMS), the *State Trait Anxiety Inventory (STAI)* – and gave us a sample of salivary cortisol. They then received their standardized 45-minute massage (see below). After the massage, they completed their rating of the massage and gave us a saliva sample. Finally, they completed the STAI and the POMS again. The immune measures were selected as being important for cellular immunity, including natural killer cell cytotoxicity, the CD3, CD4 and CD8 markers, natural killer cells with the CD56 marker, and cells expressing the CD56 but not CD3 markers. Clinically, the measures chosen were thought to be relevant for fighting off viruses and tumors (Whiteside & Herberman 1989). Measures also included those relevant in HIV disease progression – CD4 cells, CD8 cells, neopterin and beta 2 microglobulin (Lifson et al 1992). Endocrine measures included three hormones thought to be related to stress (norepinephrine, epinephrine, and cortisol), which were measured in 24-hour urine.

*Massage therapy procedure.* The 45-minute massage protocol was developed to encourage relaxation and reduction of stress. The protocol included several types of strokes (effleurage, petrissage, stroking, stretching, rocking, squeezing, and holding) on several areas of the body: in the supine position, head and neck, arms, torso, legs; in the prone position, legs and back.

**Table 6.1**  Anxiety and relaxation changes over the course of the month-long massage period (Study 1)

| | Massage – all subjects | | | |
|---|---|---|---|---|
| | Pre | Post | | |
| Variables | Mean (SD) | Mean (SD) | $n$ | $t$ |
| State Anxiety | 39.00 (10.5) | 31.89 (8.6) | 28 | 3.28** |
| POMS Anxiety | 11.20 (10.2) | 6.50 (4.2) | 20 | 2.10* |
| Relaxation | 53.79 (22.4) | 79.83 (19.0) | 29 | −5.14** |

\* $p < 0.05$; \*\* $p < 0.01$.

**Table 6.2**  Immune changes over the course of the month-long massage period (Study 1)

| | Massage – all subjects | | | | | | | |
|---|---|---|---|---|---|---|---|---|
| | Pre | Post | | | Massage positive $F$ | Massage negative $F$ | Control positive $F$ | Inter action $F$ |
| Variables | Mean (SD) | Mean (SD) | $n$ | $F$ | (Mean Δ) | (Mean Δ) | (Mean Δ) | (Mean Δ) |
| CD4 # | 519.81 (267.1) | 563.12 (391.6) | 26 | 0.22 | 0.66 | 0.04 | 1.37 | 3.10 |
| CD4/CD8 | 0.77 (0.5) | 0.77 (0.5) | 26 | 0.01 | 0.32 | 0.14 | 0.24 | 1.02 |
| Neopterin | 4.31 (4.3) | 3.54 (2.7) | 29 | 1.82 | 1.54 | 0.32 | 0.08 | 3.65 (−5.35) |
| NKH[1] # | 214.92 (161.1) | 252.20 (142.8) | 25 | 1.49 | 0.23 | 3.57 | 2.59 | 7.24* (89.45) |
| CD56 lymph | 101.71 (68.2) | 157.00 (110.8) | 24 | 7.90* | 4.04 (47.44) | 4.84 (78.83) | 2.02 | 4.97 (83.78) |
| NKH1 cytotoxicity | 24.43 (16.4) | 33.29 (19.5) | 18 | 23.23** | 23.33** (8.86) | | 7.95* (−8.05) | 16.97* (18.36) |
| CD8 # | 751.77 (328.4) | 821.46 (394.1) | 26 | 1.14 | 1.69 | 0.37 | 20.88* (−176.18) | 19.10* (369.78) |
| Soluble CD8 | 606.46 (360.6) | 812.16 (583.1) | 29 | 7.40* | 7.95* (293.03) | 0.18 | 0.61 | 0.76 |
| S6F1+CD8+ # | 686.55 (338.9) | 881.18 (437.4) | 11 | 5.02* | 5.02* (194.63) | | 1.23 | 8.18* (274.38) |

\* $p < 0.05$; \*\* $p < 0.01$.

## Results

Although anxiety decreased and relaxation increased, the massage did not affect the immune measures related to disease progression in HIV. However during the massage period there was a significant increase in NK cytotoxicity (see Tables 6.1 and 6.2). The number of NK cells as defined by CD56 decreased during the control period, and increased during the massage period. Urinary cortisol decreased during the massage period and increased during the control period. Each of the psychological (anxiety, relaxation rating) and neuroendocrine (cortisol) measures which changed significantly (Table 6.3) during the massage period were correlated with the significant immune measure changes.

The importance of the maintenance of natural killer cell number and natural killer cell cytotoxicity in HIV-positive persons is twofold. First, since HIV destroys CD4 cells, the NK cells are another type of immune cell that may substitute for the CD4 cells. In later stages of HIV infection, it has been hypothesized that in persons with low CD4 counts, those who remain asymptomatic may have greater NK cell function (Solomon et al 1993). Second, NK cells are supposed to provide protection against both viruses and tumors (Whiteside & Herberman 1989). NK cytotoxicity may be important in other diseases, such as cancer. Lower NK activity is associated with the development of metastases and shorter survival time in patients with cancer (see Whiteside & Herberman, 1989 for a review).

Given that elevated stress hormones (catecholamines and cortisol) negatively affect immune function, the increase in NK activity probably derived from the decrease in these stress hormones following massage therapy. Because NK cells are the front line of

**Table 6.3** Neuroendocrine changes over the course of the massage and control periods (Study 1)

| | Massage positive | | | Control | |
| | Pre | Post | | Positive | Interaction |
| Variables | Mean (SD) | Mean (SD) | $F$ | $F$ | $F$ |
|---|---|---|---|---|---|
| Norepinephrine µg/24 h | 31.19 (13.2) | 26.45 (16.9) | 0.49 | 0.32 | 0.25 |
| Epinephrine µg/24 h | 6.30 (4.9) | 3.43 (3.0) | 2.02 | 0.01 | 0.29 |
| Cortisol µg/24 h | 44.09 (26.7) | 23.51 (19.0) | 5.52* | 4.12 | 11.22* |

* $p < 0.05$.

defense in the immune system, combating the growth and prolif-eration of viral cells, the HIV patients who received the massage therapy would probably experience fewer opportunistic infections such as pneumonia and other viruses that often kill them. Inasmuch as NK cells are also effective in combating cancer cells, cancer patients might also benefit from massage therapy.

# CANCER

## Study 2: Massage therapy for breast cancer

Breast cancer is one of the most common cancers among women, striking one in every nine women (National Cancer Institute 1995). Although breast cancer treatment depends on many factors (e.g., stage of disease, age, menopausal status, and overall health), stan-dard procedures include surgery (lumpectomy, partial or total mas-tectomy) followed by chemotherapy, hormonal or radiation therapy.

Women diagnosed with breast cancer often suffer from *depression* and *anxiety* (Ingram 1990). Biofeedback and/or cognitive therapy e.g., progressive muscle relaxation, stress and coping training, guided imagery) appear to stabilize, but not reduce, cortisol, stress and anxiety levels (Gruber et al 1993), improve overall mood state, and decrease pain perception in some cases (Arathuzik 1991). In one study, an intervention that included EMG biofeedback train-ing, guided imagery and relaxation training was found to corre-late with significant changes in natural killer cell number and activity (Gruber et al 1993).

Massage therapy has also been found to increase natural killer cell number and activity, although it has not yet been studied with cancer patients. In the massage therapy study with HIV men just reviewed, the men received daily massages for 1 month and for the other month they did not (Ironson et al 1996). During the month of massage, increases occurred in natural killer cell number and natural killer cell cytotoxicity (activity). Natural killer cells are thought to ward off cancer cells as well as viral cells, making massage therapy a potentially effective intervention for cancer patients. Massage therapy has also been shown to decrease anxiety and depression, and lower stress hormones (cortisol) and cate-cholamines (norepinephrine/epinephrine) (Field et al 1996). Decreased stress hormones such as cortisol may contribute to enhanced immune function since cortisol is noted to destroy immune cells.

The present study was designed to explore massage therapy effects on (1) boosting the immune system by increasing natural killer cell number and cytotoxicity and (2) enhancing psychological status by reducing depression and anxiety. Because massage therapy has been effective with numerous physical and psychological conditions associated with breast cancer (anxiety, depression, elevated stress and stress hormones, compromised immune system, and pain), massage therapy was also expected to reduce these problems in breast cancer patients.

## Method

**Subjects** The sample was comprised of 20 women diagnosed with Stage I or II breast cancer who had undergone simple mastectomy (the removal of a breast) within the past one and a half years (mean age = 52.2). Subjects were middle socioeconomic status (mean = 2.0 on the Hollingshead two-factor index) and varying ethnicity (21% Hispanic and 79% Caucasian). Because radiation therapy affects immune measures, subjects were not entered into the study until completion of their radiation and chemotherapy treatment, which lasted for 6–7 weeks following surgery.

**Procedures** Subjects were randomly assigned to a body-massage ($N$=10), or to a control group ($N$=10).

*Body-massage therapy.* These were 30-minute sessions conducted by massage therapists two times a week for five consecutive weeks to alleviate stress, anxiety and depression. The therapy, comprised of Swedish massage techniques using moderate pressure and smooth stroking, covered the head/neck, shoulders, chest, arms, legs and back.

**Assessments**

*Immediate effects (pre/post-session measure).* On the first and last days of the 5-week study, pre and post the massage sessions, control subjects were asked to complete the following questionnaires: (1) *State Trait Anxiety Inventory (STAI)* (Spielberger et al 1970); (2) *Profile of Mood States Depression Scale* (POMS) (McNair et al 1971); (3) *Short-Form McGill Pain Questionnaire* (SF-MPQ) (Melzack 1987); (4) *Visual analogue scale* (VAS) (Melzack 1987).

*Longer-term effects (first/last day measures).* On the first and last days of the 5-week study, just prior to the sessions, subjects were asked to complete several questionnaires:

1. *Symptom Checklist-90RR* (SCL-90–R, Derogatis 1983) measures depression, anxiety, and hostility on a 5-point scale ranging from (0) not at all to (4) extremely. Subjects respond to how distressed they felt over the past week on depression items (e.g., 'crying easily', 'loss of sexual interest or pleasure'), anxiety (e.g., 'heart pounding or racing' 'feeling tense or keyed up') and hostility (e.g.,

'shouting or throwing things', 'having urges to break or smash things'). This inventory has high internal consistency (mean coefficient = 0.84) and test–retest reliability (mean coefficient = 0.84) and acceptable construct validity.

2. *Functional Assessment of Cancer Therapy Scale* (FACT–B, Brady et al 1997) is a 44-item self report that measures quality of life in breast cancer patients. The subscales are physical well-being, social/family well-being, relationship with doctor, emotional well-being, functional well-being and additional concerns. Participants answer how true each statement has been for them during the past week on a scale of (0) not at all to (4) very much. A characteristic statement for each subscale includes 'I have a lack of energy,' 'I feel distant from my family', 'I have confidence in my doctor', 'I worry that my condition will get worse', 'I am able to work (including work in home)', and 'I am able to feel like a woman'. This scale has been demonstrated to have high internal consistency (alpha = 0.90) and acceptable test–retest reliability.

*Biochemical measures.* On the morning of the first and the last day of the 5-week study, the participant was asked to refrain from eating or drinking and to provide a urine sample. This sample was logged, frozen and sent to Duke University for assaying of endocrine stress measures (norepinephrine, epinephrine and cortisol) and urinary 5-HIAA, a metabolite of serotonin and a marker of depression. Norepinephrine, epinephrine and serotonin assays were conducted using HPLC–ECD techniques. Urinary cortisol was determined by RIA methodology using a 125I-labeled kit (Diagnostic Products Corp., Los Angeles, Ca) following instructions provided by the supplier. Based on previous massage therapy findings, norepinephrine, epinephrine and cortisol values were expected to decrease (Field, Grizzle et al 1996; Ironson et al 1996) and 5-HIAA was expected to increase (Field et al 1996, Field, Hernandez-Reif et al 1998).

*Immune measures.* Subsequent to providing a urine sample, the participant had her blood drawn to assay immune measures relevant to cellular immunity that fight off tumors and viruses (Whiteside & Herberman 1989). The selected measures were: *Natural killer cell number and cytotoxity (NKCC).* These were assayed using the whole blood chromium release assay. NK sensitive erythroleukemia K562 cell-line was used as the target cell line. The assays were done in triplicate at four target to effector cell ratios with a 4 hour incubation. Natural killer cells are thought to fight off viruses and tumors. Increased natural killer cell number, natural killer cell cytotoxicity, soluble CD8, and the cytotoxic subset of CD8 cells were found in HIV positive men following one-month of daily massage therapy sessions (Ironson, Field et al 1996).

*Results*

**Data analyses** Repeated measures multivariate analysis of variance tests were performed on the (1) *short-term measures* (STAI, POMS), (2) the *longer-term self reports* (SCL-90–R), (3) the *biochemical urinary measures* (norepinephrine, epinephrine, cortisol and serotonin) and (4) the *immune measures* (natural killer cell number and cytotoxicity). The repeated measures were sessions (pre/post treatment or control period) and days (first/last day of the study). Significant interaction effects were followed by alpha corrected *t*-tests.

*Immediate effects (pre/post-session measure).* A significant group by sessions interaction effect for the STAI suggested that anxiety was reduced for the massage therapy group after the first and the last session (see Table 6.4). A significant group by sessions interaction effect for the POMS depression score and for the POMS anger score revealed a reduction in depressed and angry mood for the massage therapy group after the first and last sessions.

*Longer term effects (first/last day).* A days by group interaction effect for the symptom checklist (SCL-90–R) confirmed less depressive symptoms for the massage therapy group by the last day of the study. And a days by group interaction effect, $F(1, 15) = 5.63$, $p < 0.05$, suggested improved quality of life for the massage therapy group, reflected by self-reports of less distress with cancer concerns (see Table 6.5).

*Immune measures.* A significant group by days MANOVA effect on the immune measures, $F(8, 11), = 3.74, p < 0.05$, and subsequent t-tests revealed an increase in CD3+ cells, CD11a+ cells, NKH1+

**Table 6.4** Means (and standard deviations in parentheses) for the massage therapy and control group for immediate effects (pre/post session) on first and last days (Study 2)

| | Massage group | | | | Control group | | | |
|---|---|---|---|---|---|---|---|---|
| | First day | | Last day | | First day | | Last day | |
| Variables | Pre | Post | Pre | Post | Pre | Post | Pre | Post |
| *Immediate effects* | | | | | | | | |
| Anxiety (STAI) | 39 (17)$_a$ | 30 (16)$_b$** | 39 (11)$_a$ | 29 (7)$_b$** | 32 (6)$_a$ | 31 (6)$_a$ | 35 (12)$_a$ | 31 (7)$_a$ |
| Mood (POMS) | | | | | | | | |
| Depression | 15 (11)$_a$ | 8 (11)$_b$** | 10 (7)$_b$* | 7 (8)$_b$* | 4 (5)$_a$ | 4 (5)$_a$ | 8 (11)$_a$ | 6 (10)$_a$ |
| Anger | 12 (7)$_a$ | 3 (4)$_b$** | 8 (7)$_b$* | 4 (4)$_a$* | 5 (6)$_a$ | 5 (8)$_a$ | 5 (8)$_a$ | 6 (7)$_a$ |
| Vigor | 21 (7)$_a$ | 20 (4)$_a$ | 18 (7)$_a$ | 19 (5)$_a$ | 19 (4)$_a$ | 19 (5)$_a$ | 18 (6)$_a$ | 20 (6)$_a$ |

* Lower numbers are optimal for all variables. Different letter subscript indicates differences for adjacent numbers whereas superscripts indicate significance levels for those differences. Values appearing in column 3 (within groups) reflect the differences between pre/first versus pre/last days (* $p < 0.05$, ** $p < 0.01$).

cells, and the lymphocyte CD56+:CD3–CD8– cells for the massage therapy group (see Table 6.6). The control group showed a decrease in lymphocyte CD56+:CD8+CD3+ and NK CD56+:CD3–CD8– by the last day of the study.

## Discussion

Massage therapy reduced anxiety and depressed mood in our sample of women with breast cancer. Similar findings following

**Table 6.5** Means (and standard deviations in parentheses) for the massage therapy and control group for longer-term (first/last days) measures (Study 2)

| | Massage group | | Control group | |
|---|---|---|---|---|
| Variables | First day | Last day | First day | Last day |
| *Symptom checklist (SCL-90–R)* | | | | |
| Depression | 15 (9)$_a$ | 9 (7)$_b$** | 6 (4)$_a$ | 9 (10)$_a$ |
| Anxiety | 4 (3)$_a$ | 1 (2)$_b$ | 3 (3)$_a$ | 4 (3)$_a$ |
| Hostility | 5 (4)$_a$ | 2 (2)$_b$* | 3 (3)$_a$ | 3 (3)$_a$ |
| *Quality of life (FACT–B)* | | | | |
| Physical | 4 (2)$_a$ | 3 (2)$_a$ | 2 (2)$_a$ | 4 (3)$_a$ |
| Social | 19 (5)$_a$ | 19 (5)$_a$ | 24 (2)$_a$ | 23 (3)$_a$ |
| Doctor | 7 (1)$_a$ | 7 (1)$_a$ | 7 (2)$_a$ | 7 (2)$_a$ |
| Emotional | 5 (3)$_a$ | 5 (4)$_a$ | 3 (2)$_a$ | 4 (3)$_a$ |
| Functional | 19 (4)$_a$ | 20 (5)$_a$ | 25 (3)$_a$ | 25 (3)$_a$ |
| Other concerns | 14 (5)$_a$ | 10 (4)$_b$* | 14 (4)$_a$ | 14 (5)$_a$ |

A lower score is optimal. Different letter subscripts indicate differences between adjacent columns. Superscripts indicate significance levels (* $p < 0.05$, ** $p < 0.01$).

**Table 6.6** Means (and standard deviations in parentheses) for the massage therapy and control group for immune measures on first and last days

| | Massage group | | Control group | |
|---|---|---|---|---|
| Variables | First day | Last day | First day | Last day |
| CD56+ cells | 228 (146)$_a$ | 210 (122)$_a$ | 224 (88)$_a$ | 205 (62)$_a$ |
| CD3+ cells | 1162 (383)$_a$ | 1283 (425)$_a$** | 1084 (364)$_a$ | 1185 (352)$_a$ |
| CD11a+ cells | 513 (282)$_a$ | 572 (319)$_b$* | 434 (207)$_a$ | 489 (146)$_a$ |
| NKH1+ cells | 219 (67)$_a$ | 278 (108)$_b$* | 260 (96)$_a$ | 236 (74)$_a$ |
| Lymphocyte markers | | | | |
| CD56+:CD3– | 195 (108)$_a$ | 214 (86)$_a$ | 166 (79)$_a$ | 152 (70)$_a$ |
| CD56+:CD8+CD3+ | 41 (33)$_a$ | 41 (26)$_a$ | 56 (55)$_a$ | 40 (39)$_b$* |
| CD56+:CD8–CD3– | 105 (53)$_a$ | 132 (61)$_b$* | 110 (46)$_a$ | 89 (48)$_b$* |
| NK activity | | | | |
| CD56+:CD3– | 34 (13)$_a$ | 31 (13)$_a$ | 36 (14)$_a$ | 34 (14)$_a$ |
| CD56+:CD3–CD8– | 40 (17)$_a$ | 36 (14)$_a$ | 50 (22)$_a$ | 41 (19)$_a$ |

* Higher values are optimal. Different letter subscripts reflect differences for adjacent columns (* $p < 0.05$, ** $p < 0.01$).

massage therapy have been reported for other chronic illnesses including HIV (Ironson et al 1996), multiple sclerosis (Hernandez-Reif, Field et al 1998) and the autoimmune diseases of fibromyalgia (Sunshine, Field et al 1996) and chronic fatigue syndrome (Field, Sunshine et al 1997). This might also explain why the women who received massage therapy reported less angry mood and hostile symptoms.

Women in the massage therapy group also showed an increase in 5-HIAA levels, a serotonin metabolite that has been negatively correlated with depression. These optimal changes in the self-reports and biochemical measures concur with other studies on massage therapy effects for anxious and depressed moods (Field, Grizzle et al 1996; Field, Morrow et al 1992).

The critical finding that 5-weeks of massage therapy was sufficient to positively alter immune function in the women with breast cancer is compelling. First, these findings provide evidence of the study's external validity as they concur with the finding of enhanced immune function in men with HIV following massage therapy (Ironson et al 1996). Second, the increase in NKH1 cells in the breast cancer women receiving massage therapy is encouraging since a possible role for NK cells is immunosurveillance against developing tumors (Abbas et al 1991).

The mechanism underlying the improvement in immune function may be related to the decrease in cortisol levels, as cortisol stress hormones are suspected of destroying immune cells. Taken together, these findings could result in an improvement in quality of life and perhaps longer survival rate.

Further research is needed to examine whether extended massage therapy (e.g. over 6-months) can keep the cancer in remission. In addition, two massages a week may be as cost-effective as three massages a week. In our first study, daily massages over one-month were shown to enhance immune function while the present study showed positive findings with one-fourth less massage time.

## Study 3: Pediatric oncology patients benefit from massage therapy

Cancer treatment involves acute distress for children, generally caused by (1) anxiety and pain associated with medical procedures, such as bone marrow aspirations, lumbar and venous punctures and chemotherapy, and (2) nausea and vomiting resulting from chemotherapy and from conditioned anxiety associated with treatment. These repeated procedures may lead to symptoms such as anxiety, withdrawal, insomnia, nightmares, and depression.

The potential benefits of relaxation therapy have been explored for stress management. For example, relaxation training has been noted to reduce stress and enhance endorphin production in depressed adolescents (Reynolds & Coats 1986), to reduce anxiety, heart rate and cortisol levels and increase positive affect in depressed children (Platania-Solazzo et al 1992), and to reduce pain in leukemic patients (Pederson 1996). Progressive muscle relaxation has been reported to reduce feelings of nausea and anxiety induced by chemotherapy in cancer patients (Arakawa 1997).

Benefits have been demonstrated by other forms of psychological interventions. In a study evaluating the distress levels in children with leukemia, the parents noted the child had a lower level of distress using a combination of pharmacological and psychological interventions (Kazak et al 1996). One study reported the use of cognitive behavioral techniques from both parent and child as instruments to improve positive mood during painful procedures. Imagery using visualization has also led to less distress behavior during painful procedures such as children undergoing cardiac catheterization (Pederson 1995).

Massage therapy is another effective stress management procedure used to reduce pain, for example, in juvenile rheumatoid arthritis (Field et al 1996) and to reduce distress during painful procedures (Scafidi et al 1986) and postoperative pain (Nixon et al 1997). Massage has also reduced anxiety, depression and stress hormones (norepinephrine and cortisol) as well as improved sleep in child and adolescent psychiatric patients (Field et al 1992). Finally, as already noted, massage has enhanced immune function (increased number of natural killer cells and NK cell cytotoxicity) in HIV men (Ironson et al 1996) and in breast cancer women (Hernandez-Reif et al 1999) suggesting that massage therapy positively affects the immune system. Natural killer cells are noted to ward off viral and cancer cells, highlighting the potential value of massage for children with cancer (Whiteside & Herberman 1989).

The present study assessed the effects of massage therapy on the behavior, physiology, and immune function of children diagnosed with cancer. The parents were taught to give the massage therapy so that it could be given on a daily basis, could be cost-effective and might reduce the parents' stress. For example, anxiety and cortisol levels have been reduced in elderly volunteers through giving children massage (Field et al 1996). Massage therapy was expected to reduce stress and enhance immune function in the children. In addition, we hoped to reduce the oversensitivity to physical touch often noted in these children. Finally, massage was the preferred therapy because other relaxation therapy techniques require more active participation and understanding by the participant. Teaching the parents to massage their child was expected to give the parents a more active role in their child's treatment, thereby reducing their own anxiety levels and sense of helplessness. Having the parents massage the children at home was also less likely to cause an association between massage and any painful, uncomfortable medical procedures at the hospital. In addition, having the parents as therapists was considered more cost effective and potentially helpful for the parent–child relationship.

## Methods

**Sample** Twenty children with cancer (mean age = 7.2) participated in this study. The parents were middle class (mean = 2.0 on the Hollingshead) and distributed 67% Caucasian, 20% White Hispanic, and 13% Black. A majority of the children (90%) had been diagnosed with leukemia. The children, referred by the Pediatric Oncologist or child Life Specialists from the Oncology ward, were randomly assigned to the massage or control group based upon a stratification procedure to ensure baseline equivalence between groups. The groups did not differ on the above variables.

### Procedures

*Standard medical care.* During the study period, all cancer patients continued to receive standard medical care, which included examinations by a pediatric oncologist, radiation or chemotherapy and other medical procedures.

*Massage therapy group.* On the first day of the study, the parent who elected to participate was trained to give the massage. They were told that the massage was expected to help the child relax and could be used to reduce stress prior to medical procedures. The training sessions were conducted by two massage therapists. The parents were guided through the 20-minute massage by having them practice it on their child under the direction of the therapist. Once they felt comfortable doing the massage, the parents were instructed to give the massage before bedtime every day for 30 days. The 20-minute massage consisted of applying moderate pressure for 30-second periods on the face, neck, shoulders, back, stomach, legs, feet, arms and hands.

The control group parents were visited by the researcher and asked to complete the questionnaires on the first and last weeks of the study.

**Assessments** The parents completed questionnaires on their anxiety, mood, depression, personal coping with the child's condition, and their perception of their child's tactile sensitivity and distress during IV placement. Anxiety, mood and depression were also assessed for the child.

*Pre/post-session assessments (immediate effects).* These assessments were made before and after the massage sessions on the first and last days of the 30-day study.

1. *Parent assessments*:
(a) *The State Anxiety Inventory for Children* (STAIC) (Spielberger 1973)
(b) *Profile of Mood States* (POMS)
(c) *Happy Face Scale* and
(d) *Biochemical measures* – saliva samples for cortisol assays were collected at the beginning of the therapy sessions and 20 minutes after the end of the sessions.

*First/last day assessments (long-term effects)*

1. *Parent assessments*:
(a) *Effects of child's cancer on the parent and family.* This 9-item scale was designed specifically for this study. Using a 5-point scale ranging from 1 = never to 5 = always, parents answered questions on the impact of the child's cancer on discipline, tension in the home, social activities of the family, parents' sleep and daily routine.
(b) *Coping Index.* On this 24-item scale parents rated their child's anxiety, soothability and stability and their own coping on Likert Scales ranging from 'Not at all' characteristic (0) to 'All of the time' (4).
(c) *Center for Epidemiological Studies Depression Scale* (CESD, Radloff, 1977) as already described.

2. *Child assessments by parent*:
(a) *Tactile Defensiveness Scale* (Appendix 5A)
(b) *Child's IV Placement Distress Behaviors* (Elliot et al 1993). Parents were asked to record distress behaviors that occurred during the most recent IV placement procedure. The categories were:

   (i) *information seeking* – the child asks questions regarding medical procedure
   (ii) *crying* – the child displays tears and/or low pitched nonword sounds of more than 1-second duration
   (iii) *screaming* – the child expresses loud, nonword, shrill vocal expressions at high pitch intensity

(iv) *physical restraint* – child is physically restrained with noticeable pressure and/or child is exerting bodily force and resistance in response to restraint

(v) *verbal resistance* – child expresses intelligible verbal expressions of delay, termination, or resistance

(vi) *seeking emotional support* – child displays verbal or non-verbal solicitation of hugs, physical or verbal comfort from parents or staff

(vii) *verbal pain* – child says any words, phrases, or statements in any tense that refer to pain or discomfort

(viii) *flailing* – child displays random gross movement of arms, legs, or whole body. The parents also recorded the severity of behavioral distress as: mild, moderate, or severe.

3. *Child assessments*:

(a) Center for Epidemiological Studies Depression Scale (CES–D) (Radloff 1977)

(b) Complete Blood Count (CBC). The immune measures were collected from the blood work on the first and last days of the study from the patient's medical file. The complete blood count, comprised of the white blood cell count, platelet count, red blood cell count, and hemoglobin level, was examined to see if the child was in the normative range to continue treatment.

### Results

Data analyses revealed that the parents and children were less anxious after the massage sessions and the children were less distressed by the medical procedures by the end of the study (see Table 6.7). The children became less tactile defensive and less depressed. Finally, the children improved on all blood count measures including white blood cell count, platelet count, red blood cell count, and hemoglobin level.

### Discussion

The reduction of anxiety in parents of these children may have resulted from their having a more active role in their children's treatment. The children's lower anxiety following massage may have in turn contributed to their greater ability to cooperate with the medical procedures. Lower anxiety and stress hormones in the previous study on women with breast cancer was related to enhanced immune function. Reduced anxiety may have also contributed to improved immune function in these children.

**Table 6.7** Child and parent assessments for massage group (Study 3)

| Variable | First day mean | Last day mean | t | p | Optimal score |
|---|---|---|---|---|---|
| *Child assessments* | | | | | |
| IV placement | 4.0 | 5.0 | 1.73 | 0.18 | high |
| Anticipation | 1.8 | 4.3 | 1.22 | 0.32 | high |
| Procedure | 4.8 | 3.0 | 4.56 | 0.05 | low |
| Fear | 3.8 | 4.5 | 1.57 | 0.21 | high |
| CES–D | 30.0 | 29.8 | | 0.95 | low |
| Child Coping | 9.3 | 9.3 | | 1.0 | low |
| Making Child Cope | 8.7 | 7.7 | | 0.42 | low |
| Child Coping Response | 7.0 | 7.0 | | 1.0 | low |
| *Parent assessments* | | | | | |
| Cancer feelings | 18.3 | 18.3 | | 1.0 | low |
| Cancer Questionnaire | 7.0 | 6.0 | | 0.22 | low |
| Parent Coping Index | 49.3 | 41.3 | | 0.46 | low |

REFERENCES

Abbas AK, Lichtman AH, Pober JP 1991 Cellular and molecular immunology. Philadelphia, PA: WB Saunders Co

Arakawa S 1997 Relaxation to reduce nausea, vomiting, and anxiety induced by chemotherapy in Japanese patients. Cancer 20:342–349

Arathuzik MD 1991 The appraisal of pain and coping in cancer patients. Western Journal of Nursing Research 13:714–731

Brady M, David C, Mo F et al 1997 Reliability and validity of the functional assessment of cancer therapy–breast quality of life instrument. Journal of Clinical Oncology 15:974–986

Derogatis L 1983 Symptom Checklist-90–Reused. Administration, scoring and procedural manual II. Clinical Psychometric Research 19:201–209

Diego M, Jones NA, Field T, Hernandez-Reif M, Schanberg S, Kuhn C, McAdam V, Galamaga R, Galamaga M 1998 Aromatherapy reduces anxiety and enhances EEG patterns associated with positive mood and alertness. International Journal of Neuroscience 96:217–224

Elliot C, Jay S, Woody P 1993 An observation scale for measuring children's distress during medical procedures. In: Roberts M, Kocher G (eds) Readings in pediatric psychology. New York (NY): Plenum Press

Fawzy FI, Kemeny ME, Fawzy NW, Elashoff R, Morton D, Cousins N, Fahey JJ 1990 A structured psychiatric intervention for cancer patients. Archives of General Psychiatry 47:729–735

Field T, Grizzle N, Scafidi F 1996 Massage and relaxation therapies' effects on depressed adolescent mothers. Adolescence 31:903–911

Field T, Hernandez-Reif M, Quintino O, Schanberg S, Kuhn C 1998 Elder retired volunteers benefit from giving massage therapy to infants. Journal of Applied Gerontology 17:229–239

Field T, Hernandez-Reif M, Seligman S, Krasnegor J, Sunshine W, Rivas-Chacon T, Schanberg S, Kuhn C 1996 Juvenile rheumatoid arthritis: benefits from massage therapy. Journal of Pediatric Psychology 22:607–617

Field T, Morrow C, Valdeon C, Larson S, Kuhn C, Schanberg S 1992 Massage reduces anxiety in child and adolescent psychiatric patients. Journal of the American Academy of Child and Adolescent Psychiatry 31:124–131

Field T, Sunshine W, Hernandez-Reif M, Quintino O, Schanberg S, Kuhn C, Burman I 1997 Massage therapy effects on depression and somatic symptoms in chronic fatigue syndrome. Journal of Chronic Fatigue Syndrome 3:43–51

Gruber BL, Hersh SP, Hall NR, Waletzky LR, Kunz JF, Carpenter JK, Kverno KS, Weiss SM 1993 Immunological responses of breast cancer patients to behavioral interventions. Biofeedback & Self-regulation 18:1–22

Hernandez-Reif M, Field T, Ironson G, Weiss S, Katz G (1999, unpublished data). Breast cancer patients' immune functioning (data collected at the Touch Research Institute, examining massage therapy effects on Natural Killer Cell numbers and functioning, stress hormones, and stress for women with Breast Cancer)

Hernandez-Reif M, Field T, Theakston H 1998 Multiple sclerosis patients benefit from massage therapy. Journal of Bodywork and Movement Therapies. (in press)

Ingram MA 1990 Psycho-social aspects of breast cancer. Journal of Applied Rehabilitation Counseling 20:23–27

Ironson G, Friedman A, Klimas N, Antoni M, Fletcher MA, LaPerrier A, Simoneau J, Schneiderman N 1994 Distress, denial, and low adherence to behavioral interventions predict faster disease progression in gay men infected with immunodeficiency virus. International Journal of Behavioral Medicine 1(1):90–105

Ironson G, Field T, Scafidi F, Kumar M, Patarca R, Price A, Goncalves A, Hashimoto M, Kumar A, Burman I, Tetenman C, Fletcher MA 1996 Massage therapy is associated with enhancement of the immune system's cytotoxic capacity. International Journal of Neuroscience 84:205–218

Kazak A, Blackall G, Boyer B, Brophy P, Buzaglo J, Penati B, Himelstein B 1996 Implementing a pediatric leukemia intervention for procedural pain: The impact on staff. Families, Systems & Health 14:43–56

Kiecolt-Glaser JK, Glaser R, Williger D, Stout J, Messick G, Sheppard S, Ricker D, Romisher SC, Briner W, Bonnell G, Donnerberg R 1985 Psychosocial enhancement of immunocompetence in a geriatric population. Health Psychology 4:25–41

Larson K 1982 The sensory history of developmentally delayed children with and without tactile defensiveness. American Journal of Occupational Therapy 36:590–596

Lifson AR, Hessol NA et al 1992 Serum beta 2-microglobulin and prediction of progression to IADS in HIV infection. Lancet 339:1436–1440

McNair D, Lorr M, Droppleman L 1981 EITS Manual for the Profile of Mood States. San Diego, Educational and Industrial Testing Service.

McNair DM, Lorr M, Droppleman LF 1971 POMS – Profile of Mood States. San Diego, CA. Educational and Industrial Testing Service

Melzack R 1987 The Short-form McGill Pain Questionnaire. Pain 30:191–197

National Cancer Institute 1995

Nixon N, Teschendorff J, Finney J, Karnilowicz W 1997 Expanding the nursing repertory: The effect of massage in post-operative pain. Australian Journal of Advanced Nursing 14:21–26

Pederson C 1995 Children's and adolescents' experiences while undergoing cardiac catheterization. Maternal–Child Nursing Journal 23:15–25

Pederson C 1996 Promoting parental use of nonpharmacologic techniques with children during lumbar punctures. Journal of Pediatric Oncology Nursing 17:21–20

Platania-Solazzo A, Field T, Blank J et al 1992 Relaxation therapy reduces anxiety in child and adolescent psychiatric patients. Journal of American Academy of Child and Adolescent Psychiatry 31:125–131

Radloff L 1977 The CES–D scale: A self-report depression scale for research in the general population. Applied Psychological Measures 1:385–401

Reynolds WM, Coats KI 1986 A comparison of cognitive-behavioral therapy and relaxation training for the treatment of depression in adolescents. Journal of Consulting & Clinical Psychology 54:653–660

Scafidi F, Field T, Schanberg S, Bauer C, Vega-Lahr N, Garcia R, Poirier J, Nystrom G, Kuhn C 1986 Effects of tactile/kinesthetic 'stimulation' on the clinical course and sleep/wake behavior of preterm neonates. Infant Behavior and Development 9:91–105

Solomon GF, Benton D, Harker J, Bonavida B, Fletcher MA 1993 Prolonged asymptomatic states in HIV-seropositive persons with 50 CD4+ T-Cells/mm3: Preliminary psychoimmunologic findings. Journal of Acquired Immunodeficiency Syndromes 6:1173

Spielberger C, Gorsuch R, Lushene R 1970 State-Trait Anxiety inventory manual. Palo Alto: Consulting Psychologists Press, Inc

Spielberger C 1973 State Trait Anxiety Inventory for Children. Palo Alto, CA: Consulting Psychological Press

Spielberger CD, Gorsuch RL, Lushene RE 1970 The State Trait Anxiety Inventory. Palo Alto, CA: Consulting Psychologists Press

Sunshine W, Field T, Quintino O, Fierro K, Kuhn C, Burman I, Schanberg S 1996 Fibromyalgia benefits from massage therapy and transcutaneous electrical stimulation. Journal of Clinical Rheumatology 2:18–22

Whiteside TL, Herberman RB 1989 The role of natural killer cells in human disease. Clinical Immunology and Immunopathology 53:1–23

# Summary

These, then, are the improved functions noted following massage therapy. In addition to each clinical condition being marked by unique changes, such as the increased peak air flow noted in the asthma study and the decreased glucose levels in the study on diabetes, there was also a set of common findings. Across studies, decreases were noted in anxiety, depression, stress hormones (cortisol), and catecholamines. Increased parasympathetic activity may be the underlying mechanism for these changes. The pressure stimulation associated with touch increases vagal activity, which in turn lowers physiological arousal and stress hormones (cortisol levels). The pressure is critical because light stroking is generally aversive (much like a tickle stimulus) and does not produce these effects. Decreased cortisol in turn leads to enhanced immune function. Parasympathetic activity is also associated with increased alertness and better performance on cognitive tasks. Given that most diseases are exacerbated by stress and given that massage therapy alleviates stress, receiving massages should probably be high on the health priority list along with diet and exercise.

Further research is needed, however, not only to replicate these empirical findings but also to study underlying mechanisms. Until underlying mechanisms are known, the medical community is unlikely to incorporate these therapies into practice. Thus, for example, it would be important to monitor sleep patterns and assay Substance P in pain syndromes as a potential mechanism. In addition to mechanism studies, treatment comparison studies are important not only to determine the relative effects and combined effects of different therapies such as the massage therapy combined with aromatherapy, but also the within-therapy variations such as the best massage techniques for different conditions and the arousing versus the calming effects of different types of treatment – for example, the arousing effects of rosemary and the calming effects of lavender.

## ACKNOWLEDGEMENTS

We would like to thank the parents, infants and children who participated and our colleagues who collaborated on the research. This research was supported by an NIMH Research Scientist Award (#MH00331) and an NIMH Research Grant (#MH46586) to Tiffany Field and funding from Johnson and Johnson.

# Further reading: *Touch Research Institutes studies*

## PUBLISHED ARTICLES

1. *Aromatherapy*: Adults exposed to rosemary Aromatherapy showed decreased alpha & beta EEG power suggesting increased alertness, they had lower anxiety levels and performed math computations faster. Adults exposed to lavender Aromatherapy showed increased beta power suggesting drowsiness, but were more relaxed and performed math computations faster and with fewer errors.

Diego MA, Jones NA, Field T, Hernandez-Reif M 1998 Aromatherapy reduces anxiety and enhances EEG patterns associated with positive mood and alertness. International Journal of Neuroscience 96:217–224.

2. *Asthma*: This study showed positive effects of parents massaging their asthmatic children including increased peak air flow, improved pulmonary functions, less anxiety and lower stress hormones (cortisol) in the children. Parental anxiety also decreased.

Field T, Henteleff T, Hernandez-Reif M et al 1998 Children with asthma have improved pulmonary functions after massage therapy. Journal of Pediatrics 132:854–858.

3. *Attention deficit hyperactivity disorder*: Adolescents with ADHD rated themselves as happier and were observed to fidget less after massage sessions. Also, teachers rated children receiving massage as less hyperactive and as spending more time on-task.

Field T, Quintino O, Hernandez-Reif M, Koslovsky G 1998 Attention deficit hyperactivity disorder adolescents benefit from massage therapy. Adolescence 33:103–108.

4. *Autistic children*: Touch sensitivity, attention to sounds and off task classroom behavior decreased, and relatedness to teachers increased after massage therapy.

Field T, Lasko D, Mundy P, Henteleff T, Talpins S, Dowling M 1997 Autistic children's attentiveness and responsivity improved after touch therapy. Journal of Autism & Developmental Disorders 27:333–338

5. *Bottle feeding on breast-like nipples*: Infants showed fewer stress behaviors and had greater vagal activity and more organized feeding patterns during bottle feedings using nipples that are similar to breast nipples.

Field T, Schanberg S, Davalos M, Malphurs J 1997 Bottlefeeding with a breast-like nipple. Early Child Development and Care 132:57–63.

6. *Bulimia*: Bulimic adolescent girls received massage therapy 2 times a week for 5 weeks. Effects included an improved body image, decreased depression and anxiety symptoms, decreased cortisol levels and increased dopamine and serotonin levels consistent with their lower depression.

Field T, Schanberg S, Kuhn C et al 1997 Bulimic adolescents benefit from massage therapy. Adolescence 33:131.

7. *Burn*: Massage therapy sessions given prior to debridement (skin brushing) decreased depression and anger, and the subjects appeared less anxious during behavior observations and reported less pain. Lower pulse and cortisol suggested lower stress levels.

Field T, Peck M, Krugman S, Tuchel T, Schanberg S, Kuhn C, Burman I 1997 Burn injured benefit from massage therapy. Journal of Burn Care and Rehabilitation 19:241–244.

8. *Carrying position*: Infants were carried by their mothers in soft infant carriers in face inward and face outward positions. In the face inward position they slept more and in the face outward position they were more active and interactive.

Field T, Malphurs J, Carraway K, Pelaez-Nogueras M 1996 Carrying position influences infant behavior. Early Child Development and Care 121:49–54

9. *Chronic fatigue syndrome*: Immediately following massage therapy depressed mood, anxiety and stress hormone (cortisol) levels were reduced. Following 10 days of massage therapy, fatigue related symptoms, particularly emotional stress and somatic symptoms, were reduced, as were depression, difficulty sleeping and pain.

Field T, Sunshine W, Hernandez-Reif M et al 1997 Chronic fatigue syndrome: massage therapy effects on depression and somatic symptoms in chronic fatigue syndrome. Journal of Chronic Fatigue Syndrome 3:43–51.

10. *Cocaine-exposed newborns*: The massaged newborns showed increased weight gain, better performance on the Brazelton Newborn Scale (particularly on the motor scale) and fewer postnatal complications and stress behaviors were demonstrated following massage.

Scafidi F, Field T, Wheeden A et al 1996 Cocaine-exposed preterm neonates show behavioral and hormonal differences. Pediatrics 97:851–855

11. *Cross-cultural studies of young children's touching*: Studies conducted on preschool playgrounds and at McDonald's Restaurants in Paris and Miami compared a high touch culture (France) and a low touch culture (U.S.) Data analyses suggest that preschool children in Paris are touched more by their mothers and touch each other more and are less aggressive.

Field T (In Press) Greater touch and less aggression in French versus American preschoolers. Early Child Development and Care.

12. *Cross-cultural studies on adolescent touch*: Studies were conducted in cafes and fast-food restaurants in high touch (French) and low touch (US) cultures to determine relationships between touch and aggression. Analyses of the data suggested that French adolescents touched each other more and were less aggressive.

Field T (In Press) Greater touch and less aggression in French versus American adolescents. Adolescence.

13. *Cystic fibrosis*: Children receiving daily bedtime massages from their parents reported being less anxious, and their mood and peak air flow readings improved.

Hernandez-Reif M, Field T, Krasnegor J, Martinez E 1999. Cystic fibrosis symptoms are reduced with massage therapy intervention. Journal of Pediatric Psychology 24:183–189.

14. *Dancers*: Massage therapy improved range of motion, mood, and performance (including balance and posture) and decreased stress hormone (cortisol) after one month of twice weekly massage therapy.

Hernandez-Reif M, Field T, Leivadi S et al (In Press) University dance students show increased range of motion following massage therapy. Journal of Dance Medicine & Science Psychology 24:183–189.

15. *Depressed teenage mothers*: Teenage mothers who received massage therapy versus those who received relaxation therapy were less depressed and less anxious both by their own report and based on behavior observations. In addition, their urinary cortisol levels were lower and their serotonin levels were higher, indicating they were less stressed and less depressed.

Field T, Grizzle N, Scafidi F, Schanberg S 1996 Massage and relaxation therapies' effects on depressed adolescent mothers. Adolescence 31 (124):903–911.

16. *Depressed mothers touching newborns*: Mothers with depressed symptoms were compared to mothers with non-depressed symptoms one day after delivery on how they touched their newborns following an initial feeding. Depressed mothers touched their newborns less frequently.

Lundy BL, Field T, Cuadra A, Nearing G, Cigales M, Hashimoto M 1996 Mothers with depressive symptoms touching newborns. Early Development and Parenting 5:124–130.

17. *Depressive mothers' touch*: Mothers with depressive symptoms were more likely to touch their infants in a negative way and more likely to be classified as intrusive.

Malphurs J, Raag T, Field T, Pickens J, Pelaez-Nogueras M 1996 Touch by intrusive & withdrawn mothers with depressive symptoms. Early Development and Parenting 5:111–115.

18. *Depressed mothers' infants prefer touch*: Infants showed more eye contact when adults, who were smiling and cooing also touched them as compared to infants who received smiling and cooing without touch.

Pelaez-Nogueras M, Gewirtz JL, Field T et al 1996 Infant preference for touch stimulation in face-to-face interactions. Journal of Applied Developmental Psychology 17:199–213.

19. *Depressed mothers' touching increases infants' positive affect and attention*: Depressed mothers increased their infants' positive affect and attentiveness by providing them extra touch stimulation during still-face interactions.

Pelaez-Nogueras M, Field T, Hossain Z, Pickens J 1996 Depressed mothers' touching increases infants' positive affect and attention in still-face interactions. Child Development 67:1780–1792.

20. *Dermatitis in children*: Children's affect and activity levels improved as did all measures of skin condition including less redness, lichenification, excoriation, and pruritus after massage therapy. Parents' anxiety levels also decreased.

Schachner L, Field T, Hernandez-Reif M, Duarte A, Krasnegor J 1998 Atopic dermatitis symptoms decrease in children following massage therapy. Pediatric Dermatology 15:390–395.

21. *Diabetes*: Positive effects were noted for parents massaging their children including lower parent and child anxiety and depression, and increased dietary compliance. In addition, the children's glucose levels decreased to the normal range after one month of massages.

Field T, Hernandez-Reif M, LaGreca A, Shaw K, Schanberg S, Kuhn C 1997 Massage therapy lowers blood glucose levels in children with Diabetes Mellitus. Diabetes Spectrum 10:237–239.

22. *Fibromyalgia syndrome*: Massage (as compared to transcutaneous electrical stimulation) therapy improved sleep patterns and decreased pain, fatigue, anxiety, depression and cortisol levels.

Sunshine W, Field T, Schanberg S et al 1996 Massage therapy and transcutaneous electrical stimulation effects on fibromyalgia. Journal of Clinical Rheumatology 2:18–22.

23. *Food texture*: Infants preferred pureed textures while toddlers and preschoolers preferred chunky textures. However, when infants were given experience with more complex textures, they too preferred the chunky textures.

Lundy BC, Field T, Carraway K et al 1998 Food texture preferences in infants versus toddlers. Early Child Development and Care 146:69–85

24. *Grandparent volunteers providing versus receiving massage:* Grandparent volunteers were assessed after giving infants massage for a month versus receiving massage for a month themselves. Results were: 1) they reported less anxiety and fewer depressive symptoms and an improved mood after giving infants massage; 2) their pulse decreased; 3) their cortisol levels decreased; and 4) they reported improved self esteem and a better lifestyle (e.g. fewer doctor

visits and more social contacts) after the one month period. These effects were stronger for giving infants the massages than receiving massages themselves, suggesting that the massager can benefit from simply giving massages.

Field T, Hernandez-Reif M, Quintino O, Schanberg S, Kuhn C 1998 Elder retired volunteers benefit from giving massage therapy to infants. Journal of Applied Gerontology 17:229–239.

25. *HIV-exposed newborns*: Increase in weight gain and improved performance on the Brazelton Newborn Scale (motor and state scales) were experienced by the massaged newborns.

Scafidi F, Field T 1997 HIV exposed newborns show inferior orienting and abnormal reflexes on the Brazelton Scale. Journal of Pediatric Psychology 22:105–112.

26. *HIV-positive adults*: This study examined massage therapy effects on anxiety and depression levels and on immune function. The subjects received a 45 minute massage five times weekly for a 1 month period. The findings were that: (1) anxiety, stress and cortisol levels were significantly reduced; and (2) natural killer cells and natural killer cell activity increased, suggesting positive effects on the immune system.

Ironson G, Field T, Scafidi F et al 1996 Massage therapy is associated with enhancement of the immune system's cytotoxic capacity. International Journal of Neuroscience 84:205–218.

27. *Hospital job stress*: Hospital nursing and physician staff members were provided massage therapy, relaxation therapy and music therapy. These therapies significantly reduced anxiety, depression and fatigue as well as increased vigor.

Field T, Quintino O, Henteleff, T, Wells-Keife L, Delvecchio-Feinberg G 1997 Job stress reduction therapies. Alternative Therapies in Health and Medicine 3:54–56.

28. *Infants of depressed mothers*: The infants who received massage therapy versus those who were rocked experienced: (1) greater daily weight gain; (2) more organized sleep/wake behaviors; (3) less fussiness; (4) improved sociability and soothability; (5) improved interaction behaviors and (6) lower cortisol and norepinephrine (suggesting lower stress levels) and increased serotonin (suggesting less depression).

Field T, Grizzle N, Scafidi F, Abrams S, Richardson S 1996 Massage therapy for infants of depressed mothers. Infant Behavior and Development 19:109–114.

29. *Job performance/stress*: Massaged subjects showed (1) decreased EEG alpha and beta waves and increased delta activity consistent with enhanced alertness; (2) math problems were completed in approximately half the time with approximately 50% less errors after the massage; and (3) anxiety and job stress levels were lower at the end of the 1 month period.

Field T, Ironson G, Scafidi F et al 1996 Massage therapy reduces anxiety and enhances EEG pattern of alertness and math computations. International Journal of Neuroscience 86:197–205.

30. *Juvenile rheumatoid arthritis*: Positive effects of parents massaging their arthritic children included lower anxiety and cortisol levels and less pain (particularly at night) and morning stiffness as assessed by the Parent, Child and Physician's Assessment.

Field T, Hernandez-Reif M, Seligman S et al 1997 Juvenile rheumatoid arthritis: benefits from massage therapy. Journal of Pediatric Psychology 22:607–617.

31. *Labor pain*: Massage therapy during the first fifteen minutes of each hour of childbirth decreased anxiety and pain, as well as decreased the length of labor and the need for medication.

Field T, Hernandez-Reif M, Taylor S, Quintino O, Burman I 1997 Labor pain is reduced by massage therapy. Journal of Psychosomatic Obstetrics and Gynecology 18:286–291.

32. *Learning by infants*: Touch stimulation positively affected habituation or simple learning by infants.

Cigales M, Field T, Lundy B, Cuadra A, Hart S 1997 Massage enhances recovery from habituation in normal infants. Infant Behavior & Development 20:29–34.

33. *Learning in preschoolers*: Preschoolers who received a 15-minute massage showed better performance on the block design and greater accuracy on the animal pegs subsets of the WPPSI.

Hart S, Field T, Hernandez-Reif M, Lundy B 1998 Preschoolers' cognitive performance improves following massage. Early Child Development & Care 143:59–64

34. *Migraine headaches*: Massage therapy decreased the occurrence of headaches, sleep disturbances and distress symptoms.

Hernandez-Reif M, Field T, Dieter J, Swerdlow, Diego M 1998 Migraine headaches are reduced by massage therapy. International Journal of Neuroscience 96:1–11.

35. *Multiple sclerosis*: Massage therapy decreased anxiety and depressed mood, and improved self-esteem, body image and social functioning.

Hernandez-Reif M, Field T, Theakston H 1998 Multiple Sclerosis patients benefit from massage therapy. Journal of Bodywork and Movement Therapies 2:168–174.

36. *Newborns*: Women who had extended and early contact with their newborns looked at, talked to, and touched their infants more, watched less television, and talked less on the telephone than mothers with minimal contact with their infants. These findings suggest that increased postpartum contact with infants leads not only to more interaction, but also to more touching as well as touching in more intimate places (face and head), thus highlighting the value of rooming-in arrangements for mothers and infants.

Prodromidis M, Field T, Arendt R, Singer L, Yando R, Bendell D 1995 Mothers touching newborns: a comparison of rooming-in versus minimal contact. Birth 22:196–200.

37. *Oil versus no oil massage:* Infants showed fewer stress behaviors (e.g. grimacing and clenched fists). and lower cortisol levels (stress hormones) following massage with oil versus massage without oil.

Field T, Schanberg S, Davalos M, Malphurs J 1996 Massage with oil has more positive effects on neonatal infants. Pre and Perinatal Psychology Journal 11:73–78.

38. *Post-traumatic stress disorder*: Massage therapy decreased the anxiety, depression and cortisol levels (stress hormone) of children who survived Hurricane Andrew. In addition, their drawings became less depressed.

Field T, Seligman S, Scafidi F and Schanberg S 1996 Alleviating posttraumatic stress in children following Hurricane Andrew. Journal of Applied Developmental Psychology 17:37–50.

39. *Pregnancy*: This study showed decreased anxiety and stress hormones during pregnancy and fewer obstetric and postnatal complications including lower prematurity rates following pregnancy massage.

Field T, Hernandez-Reif M, Hart S, Theakston H 1999 Pregnant women benefit from massage therapy. Journal of Psychosomatic Obstetrics and Gynecology 19

40. *Premenstrual symptoms*: Mood improved and anxiety, pain and water retention symptoms decreased with massage therapy.

Hernandez-Reif M, Martinez A, Field T, Quintino O, Hart S, Burman I (In Press) Premenstrual syndrome symptoms are relieved by massage therapy. Journal of Psychosomatic Obstetrics & Gynecology.

41. *Preterm newborns gain more weight*: Preterm infants gained 47% more weight, became more responsive, were discharged 6 days earlier at a hospital cost savings of $10,000 per infant (or 4.7 billion dollars if the 470,000 preemies born each year were massaged), and 8 months later were still showing an advantage on weight, mental and motor development. The underlying biological mechanism for weight gain in the massaged preterm newborns may

be an increased in vagal tone and, in turn, an increase in insulin (food absorption hormone).

Field T, Schanberg SM, Scafidi F et al 1986 Tactile/kinesthetic stimulation effects on preterm neonates. Pediatrics 77:654–658.

42. *Preterm infants develop better*: Preterm infants who received massage therapy as newborns showed greater weight gain and more optimal cognitive and motor development eight months later.

Field T, Scafidi F, Schanberg S 1987 Massage of preterm newborns to improve growth and development. Pediatric Nursing 13:385–387.

43. *Preterm newborns sleep better*: Preterm infants who were massaged before sleep fell asleep more quickly and slept more soundly with better sleep patterns. They showed improved weight gain as compared to infants who were not touched before sleep.

Scafidi F, Field T, Schanberg S, Bauer C, Vega-Lahr N, Garcia R 1986 Effects of tactile/kinesthetic stimulation on the clinical course and sleep/wake behavior of preterm neonates. Infant Behavior and Development 9:91–105.

44. *Preterm newborns have a better clinical course*: Preterm infants received tactile/kinesthetic stimulation over a 10-day period. The infants averaged 47% greater weight gain per day and spent more time awake and active during sleep/wake behavior observations.

Field T, Schanberg S, Bauer C et al 1990 Massage stimulates growth in preterm infants: a replication. Infant Behavior and Development 13:167–188.

45. *Psychiatric patients (child and adolescent)*: Following five 30-minute massages these children/adolescents had better sleep patterns, lower depression, anxiety and stress hormone levels (cortisol and norepinephrine) and better clinical progress.

Field T, Morrow C, Valdeon C, Larson S, Kuhn C, Schanberg S 1992 Massage therapy reduces anxiety in child and adolescent psychiatric patients. Journal of the American Academy of Child and Adolescent Psychiatry 31:125–130.

46. *Rat pups*: Maternally deprived rat pups showed increased growth hormone following simulated rubbing.

Pauk J, Kuhn C, Field T, Schanberg S 1986 Positive effects of tactile versus kinesthetic or vestibular stimulation on neuroendocrine and ODC activity in maternally deprived rat pups. Life Science 39:2081–2087.

47. *Sexual abuse*: Massage therapy reduced aversion to touch and decreased anxiety, depression and cortisol levels.

Field T, Hernandez-Reif M, Hart S et al 1997 Sexual abuse effects are lessened by massage therapy. Journal of Bodywork and Movement Therapies 1:65–69.

48. *Sleep disturbances in infants*: Infants who received massage experienced less difficulty falling asleep and better sleep patterns.

Field T, Hernandez-Reif M (In Press) Sleep problems in infants decrease following massage therapy. Early Child Development and Care.

49. *Sleep by preschoolers:* Preschool children who received massage fell asleep sooner, exhibited more restful nap time periods, had decreased activity levels and better behavior ratings.

Field T, Kilmer T, Hernandez-Reif M, Burman I 1997 Preschool Children's Sleep and Wake Behavior Improve After Massage Therapy. Early Child Development & Care 120:39–44.

50. *Smoking*: Cravings, anxious behaviors and the number of cigarettes smoked were reduced by self massage.

Hernandez-Reif M, Field T, Hart S 1999 Smoking cravings are reduced by self massage. Preventive Medicine 28:28–32.

51. *Touch in preschools*: Touch was rarely observed in infant, toddler and preschool nurseries. These data were presented to the teachers along with examples of appropriate touch, and they were requested to provide more touching in the classroom. The amount of touch subsequently increased.

Field T, Harding J, Soliday B, Lasko D, Gonzalez N, Valdeon C 1998 Touching in infant, toddler & preschool nurseries. Early Child Development and Care 98:113–120.

52. *Touch in preschoolers*: Preschool children engaged in touching behaviors demonstrated significantly less touching of vulnerable body parts than infants and toddlers. Preschoolers demonstrated less 'task' related touch but more 'communication' related touch as compared to the infants and toddlers. Affectionate touch was most prevalent among toddlers.

Cigales M, Field T, Hossain Z, Pelaez-Nogueras M, Gewirtz J 1996 Touch among children at nursery school. Early Child Development & Care 126:101–110.

# PUBLISHED REVIEWS

1. *Interventions for premature infants*: Systematic investigations of early interventions and their effects on the high-risk infant.

Field T 1986 Interventions for premature infants. Journal of Pediatrics 109:183–191.

2. *Alleviating stress in intensive-care neonates*: Intensive care nursery environments and their effects as well as positive stimulation effects are reviewed.

Field T 1987 Alleviating stress in NICU neonates. Journal of the American Osteopathic Association 87:646–650.

3. *Review of the early stimulation literature*

Schanberg S, Field T 1987 Sensory deprivation stress and supplemental stimulation in the rat pup and preterm human neonate. Child Development 58:1431–1447.

4. *Stimulation in preterm infants*: Preterm infants who received tactile stimulation showed greater weight gain. The underlying mechanism for the massage/weight gain relationship is an increase in vagal tone which in turn increases food absorption.

Field T 1988 Stimulation of preterm infants. Pediatrics in Review 10:149–154.

5. *Alleviating stress in newborns*: Intensive care nursery environments and the effects of high-intensity noise, bright lights, cold, invasive and painful procedures suggests potentially stressful effects on the newborn of which the behavioral and physiological outcomes are examined. Gentle human touch was associated with A) fewer startle responses B) decreased need for medical ventilation C) fewer clenched fists. The stimulated infants averaged greater weight gain, were awake and active for a greater period of time and scored better on the Brazelton Scale.

Field T 1990 Alleviating stress in newborn infants in the intensive care unit. Perinatology 17:1–9.

6. *Massage therapy for infants and children*: The effects of massage therapy on infants and children with various medical conditions are reviewed. The conditions range from infants who are premature, cocaine-exposed, infants of depressed mothers, HIV-exposed and infants with no medical problems. The childhood conditions include abuse (sexual and physical), asthma, burns, cancer, developmental delays, dermatitis, diabetes, eating disorders (bulimia), juvenile rheumatoid arthritis, posttraumatic stress disorder, and psychiatric disorders.

Field T 1995 Massage therapy for infants and children. Developmental and Behavioral Pediatrics 16:105–111.

7. *Massage therapy effects*: Infant, child and adult massage therapy studies ranging across many conditions are reviewed along with potential underlying mechanisms.

Field T 1998 Massage therapy effects. American Psychologist 53:1270–1281.

# STUDIES IN REVIEW

1. *Anorexia*: Massage therapy reduced anxiety and stress, and resulted in decreased body dissatisfaction associated with anorexia.

Hart S, Field T, Hernandez-Reif M, Shaw S, Schanberg S, Kuhn C (In Review) Anorexia symptoms are reduced by massage therapy. Adolescence.

2. *Autistic children*: Children with autism were massaged for one month by their parents prior to their daily bedtime. They showed increased attentiveness and less hyperactive behavior in the classroom. The massaged children also initiated positive touch more frequently when playing with their peers and showed lower fussing, crying and self stimulating behavior during sleep time.

Escalona A, Field T, Singer-Strunk R, Cullen C, Hartshorne K (In Review) Improved body image with massage therapy. Journal of Autism and Developmental Disorders.

3. *Back pain*: Massage lessened lower back pain and enhanced physical range of motion.

Hernandez-Reif M, Field T, Krasnegor J, Theakston T (In Review) Lower back pain is reduced following massage therapy. Spine.

4. *Father–infant massage*: Fathers gave their infants daily massages 15 minutes prior to bedtime for one month. The fathers in the massage group engaged more in their infant's daily caregiving tasks as well as have an improvement in the interactive behavior with the child.

Cullen C, Field T, Escalona A, Hartshorn K (In Review) Father–infant interactions are enhanced by massage therapy.

5. *Hypertension*: Massage therapy decreased diastolic blood pressure, anxiety and cortisol (stress hormone) levels.

Hernandez-Reif M, Field T, Krasnegor J, Theakston H (In Review) Hypertension symptoms are reduced by massage therapy. Psychosomatic Medicine.

6. *Post-burn*: Ten massage therapy sessions led to lower anxiety, anger, depression, pain and itching.

Field T, Peck M, Hernandez-Reif M, Krugman S, Burman I, Ozment-Schenck L (In Review) Massage therapy reduces anxiety in children with burns. Journal of Burncare and Rehabilitation.

7. *Preterm infant massage increases weight gain in five days*: Preterm infants gained more weight following only 5 days of massage therapy.

Dieter J, Field T, Hernandez-Reif M & Emory E (In Review). Preterm infants gain more weight following 5 days of massage therapy. Journal of Pediatrics.

# ONGOING STUDIES

1. *Abused and neglected children*: Massage is expected to improve caregiver infant/child interactions, to help the abused children have a less aversive response to touch and to reduce their stress levels.

2. *Aggressive adolescents*: Conduct disorder, hostility and anxiety are expected to decrease according to parental reports. In addition, the adolescents' stress hormones and testosterone levels and mood are expected to improve.

Diego M, Field T, Hernandez-Reif M (In Preparation) Effects of massage therapy on aggressive adolescents.

3. *Behavior problem children*: Preschool children with behavior problems who receive massage are expected to show more on-task behavior, less solitary play, and less aggression.

4. *Breast cancer*: Women with Stage I and II Breast Cancer who received 3 massages per week for 5 weeks reported reduced anxiety and showed increases in Natural Killer Cell numbers.

Hernandez-Reif M, Field T, Ironson G, Weiss S, Katz G (In Preparation) Breast cancer patients' immune functioning benefits from massage therapy.

5. *Carpal tunnel syndrome*: Self-administered massage therapy is expected to stretch tendons and alleviate pain.

Field T, Sunshine W, Hernandez-Reif M, Gruskin A, Burman I (In Preparation). Massage therapy reduces pain associated with carpal tunnel syndrome.

6. *Cerebral palsy*: Massage therapy is expected to help infants with CP gain more muscle flexibility, and increase posture, motor function and social interaction.

Hernandez-Reif M, Field T, Bornstein J, Fewell R (In Preparation) Cerebral palsy infants benefit from massage therapy.

7. *Colic in infants*: Infants receiving massage by their parents are expected to have more positive feeding interactions with their caregivers, be less irritable, have fewer stress behaviors and more organized sleep/wake behaviors.

8. *Coma*: Massage therapy is intended to increase serotonin and signs of alertness for children in coma.

Hernandez-Reif M, Field T & Jones N (In Preparation). Pediatric coma patients benefit from massage therapy.

9. *Couples' sex therapy*: Couples using massage prior to and during sex experiences are expected to have lower performance anxiety and increased physical intimacy.

10. *Down syndrome*: Infants with Down syndrome are expected to improve in muscle tone and in cognitive skills.

Hernandez-Reif M, Field T, Bornstein J, Fewell R (In Preparation) Enhancing motor and cognitive skills in toddlers with Down's Syndrome.

11. *HIV in adolescents*: This study is monitoring immune changes accompanying massage therapy.

12. *Irritable bowel syndrome*: Massage therapy is expected to reduce intestinal symptoms (e.g., constipation and pain) and anxiety.

13. *Parkinson patients*: Massage therapy is expected to improve cognitive skills in patients with Parkinson's disease and helps reduces anxiety.

Hernandez-Reif M, Field T, Del Pino N (In Preparation) Parkinson disease is improved by massage therapy.

14. *Pediatric oncology*: This study was designed to determine the effects of parents massaging their children with cancer. Decreased behavioral stress is expected during invasive procedures and a longer term improvement is expected in immune function.

Cullen C, Field T, Hernandez-Reif M, Sprinz P, Kissel B, Sanchez-Bango V (In Preparation) Pediatric oncology patients and their parents report reduced anxiety and improved mood following massage therapy.

15. *Preterm physiology*: Preterm newborns are receiving daily massage to study possible mechanisms underlying massage benefits including vagal activity and oxytocin levels.

Dieter JNI, Field T, Hernandez-Reif M, Redzepi M, Emory EK (In Preparation) Massage therapy effects on the physiology and behavior of preterm infants.

16. *Prostate cancer*: Men receiving massage are expected to show reduced stress hormone (cortisol) and increased immune function (natural killer cell number and activity).

17. *Sickle cell*: This study is measuring the pain alleviating effects of massage.

18. *Spinal cord injuries*: Massage therapy is expected to improve functional abilities, range of motion and muscle strength.

Diego M, Hernandez-Reif M, Field T, Brucker B, Hart S, Burman I (In Preparation) Spinal cord injury benefits from massage therapy.

19. *Sports massage*: Pre-running massage is designed to decrease anxiety and enhance alertness prior to running events.

20. *Toy texture*: This study is designed to determine the relationship between toy preferences and the texture of the toy and developmental changes in texture preferences. Texture preferences are expected to change with age, and toy preferences are expected to be associated with a texture preference.

# Appendices

# Appendix 1A
# Thermometer for feeling good

Name: _____

Date: _____

Best I have ever felt — 10

9

8

7

6

5

4

3

2

1

Not feeling good at all — 0

# Appendix 1B
# Weekend diary/checklist

*Date:*

*Time:*

*Health/exercise*
No. of hours of sleep last night          _____

No. of naps taken during the day         _____

No. of walks/exercise         _____

No. of headaches during the day        _____

Other physical complaints (please specify)      _____

No. of medications/prescriptions taken (please specify)    _____

No. of doctor's visits in the past week      _____

*Eating/drinking*
No. of cups of coffee

No. of alcoholic drinks (beer, wine, or liquor)      _____

No. of cigarettes smoked       _____

No. of meals eaten         _____

No. of meals eaten out        _____

No. of meals eaten with others       _____

No. of snacks eaten during the day      _____

*Entertainment/leisure*
No. of hours of TV watching       _____

No. of phone calls made       _____

No. of phone calls received       _____

Did you contact any family members? (please specify who) _____

No. of visitors _____

No. of sexual activities _____

No. of times hugged/kissed _____

Did you go to the hairdresser today?         yes no  _____

Did you go to the movies today?         yes no  _____

Other group activities? (please specify) _____

What did you do in your free time today? _____

*Mood state*

On a scale from 1 to 3 (1 = rarely, 2 = occasionally, 3 = frequently), please rate these mood states as they applied to your moods today:

happy
lonely
bored
depressed
anxious
scared
neutral

# Appendix 2A
# Salivary cortisol sampling

Saliva samples are collected and assayed for cortisol levels as a measure of stress. High levels of cortisol have been related to anxiety and stress. Due to a 20-minute lagtime in cortisol changes, saliva samples always reflect responses to stimulation occurring 20 minutes prior to sampling. Participants are asked to place a cotton dental swab along their gumline for 30 seconds. The swab is then placed in a syringe, and the plunger is depressed to express the saliva into a microcentrifuge tube. The saliva samples are subsequently frozen and sent to Duke University for assaying.

# Appendix 2B
# Headache history inventory

In response to each question, please circle the item(s) from one of the four columns which best describe your headaches. Please try to circle only one column's item(s) per question.

| Column 1 | Column 2 | Column 3 | Column 4 |
| --- | --- | --- | --- |
| **1. What is the severity of your headache pain?** | | | |
| Moderate or severe | Incapacitating | Mild, moderate, or severe | Mild or moderate |
| **2. How would you describe your headache pain?** | | | |
| Throbbing, pulsating, or pressure-like | Stabbing or boring | Can range from dull and nagging to throbbing, pulsating, or pressure-like | Dull, nagging or tightness |
| **3. How often do you get your headaches?** | | | |
| Can range from a few a year, to a few a month, to one or two a week. Headaches are moderate to severe. | Very severe headaches which come in cycles with months, or even years, between the cycles. | Headaches on most days of the week which range in intensity from mild to moderate or severe. | Mild pain which can occur daily, several times a week or month. |
| **4. How long do your headaches last?** | | | |
| 4–24 hours | 30–90 minutes | Often constant pain ranging from dull to moderate or severe. | Mild pain which can be of short duration to constant. |
| **5. What is the location of your headache pain?** | | | |
| Usually one side of the head. | Usually one side of the head, often in the area of the eye. | Location varies and can be on one side of the head, band-like around the head, or all over. | Both sides of the head, band-like, often including the neck. |
| **6. What are the associated symptoms of your headaches?** | | | |
| Nausea, vomiting, sensitivity to light, noise, and odors. | Flushing of face on side of pain; tearing of eye on side of pain; swelling of eyelid on side of pain; running of nose on side of pain. Sometimes dropping of eyelid on side of pain. | Nausea, vomiting, sensitivity to light, noise, order, anxiety, depression, or no associated features. | Anxiety and/or depression, or no associated features. |

# Appendix 3A
# Happy faces scale

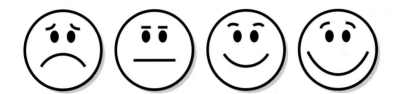

# Appendix 3B
# EEG and EKG procedures

*EEG recording*

The infant's and mother's EEG was recorded from the mid-frontal (F3 & F4) and parietal (P3 & P4) regions and referenced to the vertex (Cz). Omni-prep gel and electrode gel were inserted into each site in order to gently abrade and provide good conductance. Impedances were less than 5K ohms or the site was re-abraded until optimal impedances were obtained. The vertex reference location was used because this reference site has been shown to produce comparable results to other reference sites and it is the least invasive location for infants this age. EOG was also obtained from the outer canthus and the supro orbit position of one eye using Beckman mini-electrodes.

The EEG signals were obtained using a Grass Model 12 Neurodata Acquisition System and the output was directed to a Dell 325 D PC fitted with Analog Devices RTI-815 A/D board. The sampling rate was 512 samples per second and the data were streamed across the computer screen and then saved to a hard disk using data acquisition software (Snapstream, v. 3.21, HEM Data Corp. 1991).

*EEG analysis*

EEG data were scored for eye and motor movement artifact using the EOG channels as cues and the data containing artifact were underscored and eliminated from each channel. The data were submitted to a discrete Fourier Transform using a Hanning Window with 50% overlap. The analyses produced power for the 3–6 hertz (Hz) frequency band in picowatt ohms (one microvolt squared) for each channel which is similar to other data using the same frequency band for children of this age (Jones, Field, Fox, Lundy & Davalos, 1997). We then computed frontal and parietal asymmetry scores using the natural log power scores. The asymmetry score is a difference score reflecting the power in one hemisphere relative to the power in the contralateral hemisphere (Ln (Right)–Ln (Left)), with negative scores reflecting greater right EEG asymmetry and positive scores reflecting greater relative left EEG asymmetry.

*Vagal tone (heart rate variability)*

Vagal tone was assessed by placing 3 EKG electrodes on the infant's chest and back. The electrodes were connected to a Grass Model 12 Neurodata Acquisition system preamplifier with bandpass frequencies set at 1.0 and 100 Hz. and a gain of 2000. The output was directed to a Dell 325 D PC fitted with Analog Devices RTI-815 A/D board. The data were streamed across the computer screen at a sampling rate of 512 samples per second and then saved to a hard disk using data acquisition software (Snapstream, v. 3.21, HEM Data Corp. 1991). After scoring for artifact, EKG data were converted to inter-beat intervals (IBI) and then to vagal tone using Delta-Biometrics, Inc., Mxedit software, which utilizes an algorithm developed by Porges (1985).

REFERENCES

Jones NA, Field T, Fox NA, Davalos M, Pickens J 1997 Brain electrical activity stability in infants/children of depressed mothers. Child Psychiatry and Human Development (in press)

Porges SW 1995 Cardiac vagal tone: a physiological index of stress. Neuroscience and Biobehavioral Reviews 19:225–233

# Appendix 3C
# Life events questionnaire

*Directions*:  Please check if any of these events have happened to you within the *last four weeks*. Then rate how the event has affected your life.

|  |  | *Extremely Negative* |  |  |  |  |  | *Extremely Positive* |
|---|---|---|---|---|---|---|---|---|
| _____ | Major financial difficulties | 6 | 5 | 4 | 3 | 2 | 1 | 0 |
| _____ | Major change in health (to yourself – physical or emotional) | 6 | 5 | 4 | 3 | 2 | 1 | 0 |
| _____ | Major change in health (to family member – physical, emotional, or behavioral) | 6 | 5 | 4 | 3 | 2 | 1 | 0 |
| _____ | Major personal event (Having a baby, child getting married, formal commitment to a relationship) | 6 | 5 | 4 | 3 | 2 | 1 | 0 |
| _____ | Death of mate or lover | 6 | 5 | 4 | 3 | 2 | 1 | 0 |
| _____ | Death of other family member or close friend | 6 | 5 | 4 | 3 | 2 | 1 | 0 |
| _____ | Major difficulties in primary relationship (including divorce) | 6 | 5 | 4 | 3 | 2 | 1 | 0 |
| _____ | Relocation (>100 miles) | 6 | 5 | 4 | 3 | 2 | 1 | 0 |
| _____ | Trouble at job (fear of getting fired, conflict of values, hate it) | 6 | 5 | 4 | 3 | 2 | 1 | 0 |
| _____ | Major life decision | 6 | 5 | 4 | 3 | 2 | 1 | 0 |
| _____ | Other: _____ | 6 | 5 | 4 | 3 | 2 | 1 | 0 |

# Appendix 3D
# Job stress yesterday questionnaire

Think about what your job was like *for the past month*. Does each of the of the following words or phrases describe it?

Answer *Yes, No*, or *?* (cannot decide).　　　　　　　　How much did it bother you?

|  |  |  |  | *not at all* |  |  | *all the time* |
|---|---|---|---|---|---|---|---|
| 1. Hectic | Yes | No | ? | 0 | 1 | 2 | 3 |
| 2. Interrupted | Yes | No | ? | 0 | 1 | 2 | 3 |
| 3. Tense | Yes | No | ? | 0 | 1 | 2 | 3 |
| 4. Hassled | Yes | No | ? | 0 | 1 | 2 | 3 |
| 5. Calm | Yes | No | ? | 0 | 1 | 2 | 3 |
| 6. Relaxed | Yes | No | ? | 0 | 1 | 2 | 3 |
| 7. Comfortable | Yes | No | ? | 0 | 1 | 2 | 3 |
| 8. Overwhelming | Yes | No | ? | 0 | 1 | 2 | 3 |
| 9. Frantic | Yes | No | ? | 0 | 1 | 2 | 3 |
| 10. Pushed | Yes | No | ? | 0 | 1 | 2 | 3 |
| 11. Irritating | Yes | No | ? | 0 | 1 | 2 | 3 |
| 12. Many things stressful | Yes | No | ? | 0 | 1 | 2 | 3 |
| 13. Under control | Yes | No | ? | 0 | 1 | 2 | 3 |
| 14. Nerve-wracking | Yes | No | ? | 0 | 1 | 2 | 3 |

|  |  |  |  | *not at all* |  |  | *all the time* |
|---|---|---|---|---|---|---|---|
| 15. Pressured |  |  |  |  |  |  |  |
|  | Yes | No | ? | 0 | 1 | 2 | 3 |
| 16. Demanding |  |  |  |  |  |  |  |
|  | Yes | No | ? | 0 | 1 | 2 | 3 |
| 17. Smooth-running |  |  |  |  |  |  |  |
|  | Yes | No | ? | 0 | 1 | 2 | 3 |
| 18. More stressful than I'd like |  |  |  |  |  |  |  |
|  | Yes | No | ? | 0 | 1 | 2 | 3 |
| 19. Not enough people to do the work |  |  |  |  |  |  |  |
|  | Yes | No | ? | 0 | 1 | 2 | 3 |
| 20. Not enough time to get the work done |  |  |  |  |  |  |  |
|  | Yes | No | ? | 0 | 1 | 2 | 3 |
| 21. Heavy workload |  |  |  |  |  |  |  |
|  | Yes | No | ? | 0 | 1 | 2 | 3 |
| 22. Can't control my work schedule |  |  |  |  |  |  |  |
|  | Yes | No | ? | 0 | 1 | 2 | 3 |
| 23. Interruptions disrupt my work |  |  |  |  |  |  |  |
|  | Yes | No | ? | 0 | 1 | 2 | 3 |
| 24. Job demands too much of me |  |  |  |  |  |  |  |
|  | Yes | No | ? | 0 | 1 | 2 | 3 |
| 25. Too many things are done at once |  |  |  |  |  |  |  |
|  | Yes | No | ? | 0 | 1 | 2 | 3 |
| 26. Work never lets up |  |  |  |  |  |  |  |
|  | Yes | No | ? | 0 | 1 | 2 | 3 |
| 27. Too many things happen at once |  |  |  |  |  |  |  |
|  | Yes | No | ? | 0 | 1 | 2 | 3 |
| 28. Have to take work home |  |  |  |  |  |  |  |
|  | Yes | No | ? | 0 | 1 | 2 | 3 |
| 29. Have too much work to do |  |  |  |  |  |  |  |
|  | Yes | No | ? | 0 | 1 | 2 | 3 |
| 30. Too little time to think and plan |  |  |  |  |  |  |  |
|  | Yes | No | ? | 0 | 1 | 2 | 3 |
| 31. Too many projects at the same time |  |  |  |  |  |  |  |
|  | Yes | No | ? | 0 | 1 | 2 | 3 |

# Appendix 5A
# Tactile defensiveness scale

_____

*Teacher's name* _____     *Date* _____

*Name of child* _____

*Directions: Please circle the correct response.*

| | | | | |
|---|---|---|---|---|
| a. | This child likes to be touched | rarely | sometimes | often |
| b. | This child touches me | rarely | sometimes | often |
| c. | I touch him/her | rarely | sometimes | often |

*Directions: Please answer YES or NO.*

| | | | |
|---|---|---|---|
| 1. | Does this child avoid getting hands in fingerpaints, paste, sand, etc.? | Yes | No |
| 2. | Does this child stiffen his/her body when picked up? | Yes | No |
| 3. | Does this child seem to prefer to play alone? | Yes | No |
| 4. | Does this child enjoy playing with other children? | Yes | No |
| 5. | Does this child struggle against being held? | Yes | No |
| 6. | Does he/she rarely show a reaction to being pushed or hit by other children? | Yes | No |
| 7. | Does this child avoid using hands for an extended period of time? | Yes | No |
| 8. | Does this child dislike being held, cuddled, and hugged? | Yes | No |
| 9. | Does this child object to being touched by others? | Yes | No |
| 10. | Does he/she seem to lack awareness of being touched by others? | Yes | No |

# Appendix 5B
# Feelings about my infant/child

_____

Name of child: ————————————————  Date: ————————————

Please circle the number that *best* describes how you feel about your child.

| | Rarely | | Sometimes | | Often |
|---|---|---|---|---|---|
| 1. I really like my child | 1 | 2 | 3 | 4 | 5 |
| 2. My child gets on my nerves | 1 | 2 | 3 | 4 | 5 |
| 3. My child is demanding | 1 | 2 | 3 | 4 | 5 |
| 4. I enjoy my child | 1 | 2 | 3 | 4 | 5 |
| 5. My child gives me pleasure | 1 | 2 | 3 | 4 | 5 |
| 6. My child looks at me | 1 | 2 | 3 | 4 | 5 |
| 7. My child smiles at me | 1 | 2 | 3 | 4 | 5 |
| 8. My child makes me feel warm inside | 1 | 2 | 3 | 4 | 5 |
| 9. I like holding my child | 1 | 2 | 3 | 4 | 5 |
| 10. I have a hard time soothing my child | 1 | 2 | 3 | 4 | 5 |
| 11. My child talks to me | 1 | 2 | 3 | 4 | 5 |
| 12. I like taking care of my child | 1 | 2 | 3 | 4 | 5 |
| 13. I am patient with my child | 1 | 2 | 3 | 4 | 5 |
| 14. I like playing with my child | 1 | 2 | 3 | 4 | 5 |
| 15. I know what my child wants | 1 | 2 | 3 | 4 | 5 |
| 16. My child responds well to me | 1 | 2 | 3 | 4 | 5 |
| 17. I worry about my child's well-being | 1 | 2 | 3 | 4 | 5 |

# Index